31472400286534

SO-AWF-974

EVOLUTION
OF A REVOLUTION

EVOLUTION OF A REVOLUTION

Autism and the Path from Hope to Healing

Collected by

HELEN CONROY and **LAURA HIRSCH**

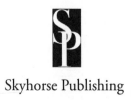

Skyhorse Publishing

Skyhorse Publishing books may be purchased in bulk at special discounts for sales promotion, corporate gifts, fund-raising, or educational purposes. Special editions can also be created to specifications. For details, contact the Special Sales Department, Skyhorse Publishing, 307 West 36th Street, 11th Floor, New York, NY 10018 or info@skyhorsepublishing.com.

Skyhorse® and Skyhorse Publishing® are registered trademarks of Skyhorse Publishing, Inc.®, a Delaware corporation.

Visit our website at www.skyhorsepublishing.com.
10 9 8 7 6 5 4 3 2 1

Library of Congress Cataloging-in-Publication Data is available on file.

Cover design by Rain Saukas
Cover photo: iStockphoto

Print ISBN: 978-1-5107-1194-5
Ebook ISBN: 978-1-5107-1195-2

Printed in the United States of America

Contents

Preface

Not very long ago, the friends behind the Thinking Moms' Revolution wanted to share the support they had found in each other and decided to write a book. That small idea became a blog, and eventually a social thought movement. TMR is known for demanding action, so it felt natural to shift from offering hope and support to offering financial assistance as well. Team TMR, a 501(c)(3) not-for-profit organization, was born. The women that contributed to this book volunteered their stories without compensation because they believe in hope, in supporting others on this path, and in the Thinking Moms' Revolution. I am awed and humbled to be in their company. When I read their stories of faith and recovery, I feel deeply connected to each of them. The funds generated from the sale of the book will benefit the Team TMR grant program and will fund treatments for children with autism and other related disorders. Thank you for supporting our mission. We remain committed to turning the tide of this epidemic, and your help is greatly appreciated.

Helen Conroy, Executive Director, Team TMR

Our goal with the Thinking Moms' Revolution was to help parents understand they are not alone. We wanted to share our stories in the hopes they would inspire others to pursue recovery with the same fervor and tenacity we did. We dared to dream that, in doing so, we would inspire a thought revolution! Along came these incredible Thinkers: moms who have done the work, some having attained the magical "R" word ("Recovery") we all strive for with each waking moment. I consider myself to be honored and blessed to be among such genuine greatness. We hope you see yourself in these pages. We hope the truth written here settles in your bones and becomes a part of you. Recovery is real. Believe it.

Lisa Joyce Goes, Board President, Team TMR

Introduction

THROUGH A VARIETY OF AVENUES, BOTH HAPPENSTANCE AND intentional, each of us at Team TMR came to know and love the Thinking Moms' Revolution. We wake up to their blog posts in our email boxes and read them over morning coffee. These mothers (and one dad) provide us with a much-needed voice, and we live vicariously through their epic adventures in the world of autism and related childhood disorders.

TMR has passed the proverbial torch, and we have been brought together and given the opportunity to share our stories of the emergence from struggle into hope and recovery. Now, the ties that bind us—to each other and to TMR—extend beyond our affected kids. We need each other like air and water. We share in each individual's successes because they might not have happened without our shared steadfast support and mountains of knowledge. The belief we hold in recovery only serves to make us stronger and make healing more realistic.

Our hope is that readers will find themselves in these pages, much in the same way we found ourselves mirrored in the Thinking Moms' Revolution. We want our stories to give you strength to keep up the fight one more day and give you the confidence to overcome this unique but shared challenge. We would like you to turn to our words when you think you just can't do it anymore. We aspire to instill in you the faith and knowledge that TMR gave us, because it was this faith and knowledge that kept us from surrendering. We believe in our very core that all children deserve to live free from physical and emotional pain in whatever way they manifest, and collectively we can make it happen.

1

Phoenix
Journey to Acceptance

"YOU ARE DOING EVERYTHING YOU CAN," SAID OUR PEDIATRICIAN when I told him of my son's autism diagnosis and confirmed that we were receiving Early Intervention services. *Everything I can.* Fifty to sixty hours of intervention services a month for a not-even-two-year-old. It wasn't helping. He was getting worse. More autistic, less the boy I knew. How could I resign myself to this, when just three months ago he was perfect? I had spent those three months getting Early Intervention services in place. A terrible agency, then a great agency, then an autism-specific agency. Months of paperwork, agonizing decisions, further regression. No progress.

Meanwhile, I was reading. I had gone to the library and taken out every book about autism they had. I didn't know anything about autism. I didn't know a single person with this diagnosis. I had no clue at that point that Andrew had about a 1-in-30 chance of becoming autistic in 2012 just by being born a boy.

I wept as I realized what had happened to my son. What I had allowed to happen. I learned about vaccines, the neurotoxins they contain, the heavy metals. But most importantly, I learned that there were things that I could do, that autism was a medical condition, and that I could improve his symptoms. I learned about biomedical treatments and diets, and later about GMOs. I convinced my husband to let us try a gluten-free diet with Andrew, just for a month, as it was expensive. I agreed that if nothing changed, I'd drop it. Just three days after eliminating gluten from Andrew's diet, we had eye contact from our sweet boy who hadn't looked at us in months, and we were hooked. There was no turning back.

Deeper and deeper I dug. As a stay-at-home mom of three, I didn't have a lot of spare time, but I was frantic to help Andrew. With every free minute, I networked, researched, and found mothers of children with autism on the same path. I was waking up, and I was very, very sad. I learned that thousands and thousands of children are sick here in the United States. You know the story now; you've read the first Thinking Moms' Revolution book. You know about vaccines, about neurotoxins, about giving Tylenol before and after shots. You know about how GMOs create holes in the stomachs of lab rats. You know about methylation mutations and the risks of vaccinating when these are present. Back then, I didn't even know about regressive autism!

According to the mainstream view, autism is something you're born with, and my son wasn't. He was born unbelievably beautiful, with a full head of dark hair and two strong cowlicks on his hairline. He was happy and healthy, and he hit every milestone either on time or early. He was the earliest crawler of my three children. Sure, he was pretty cranky as a newborn, but he always had eye contact and smiles. As soon as he was mobile, he turned into the happiest child you could hope to meet. He spoke dozens of words, he took steps. Although he wouldn't officially walk until seventeen months, he had been adeptly cruising full-time since nine months.

He was even developmentally ahead of his twin. Way ahead, actually, all along. Andrew sat at six months, Ben sat at eight months. Andrew crawled at eight months, Ben crawled at twelve months. We were actually worried about Ben, not Andrew. But there were little things I remember now about Andrew that might have been clues. One day, when all three kids were eating, Ava and Benjamin were making a lot of noise, and my mother made a comment about how Andrew never talks anymore. Or the time when we went to the park and Andrew beelined it down the hill to try to get to the stop sign across the street instead of playing on the slide. But overall, Andrew was totally under our parental worry radar.

Until he wasn't. Until we realized that he had never really fully come back to us from that 104-degree fever that lasted four days after his fifteen-month shots but that "wasn't related because he didn't have seizures." And then he was slipping away, day by day. Then, all of a sudden, Ben, who had been globally delayed all along, was doing things Andrew wasn't. We looked at each other and said, "What the hell happened here? What did we miss?"

A social worker and a speech therapist from Early Intervention, on their first trip to the house, said he was either deaf or autistic. *Deaf!* That made sense. Yes! He was deaf. That would suck, he'd have to get hearing aids and we'd all have to learn sign language, but no big deal! People who are deaf are not doomed! He could have become deaf from the high fever. He failed the regular hearing test, so we set up the sedated BAER (brainstem auditory evoked response) and prepared ourselves.

But then we realized he could hear us. Even though he didn't flinch at the loudest of noises or respond when we called his name, anytime I sang, no matter how softly, he would look for me, look at me. *Fuck.* He wasn't deaf. The BAER confirmed it two weeks before Christmas, but we'd have to wait another month for the official autism diagnosis. We still didn't know what autism was, but we knew it wasn't good, because all our family and friends had said for months was, "Better something wrong with his ears than his brain!" And that sounded right to us. Ears you can fix, brains you can't. Right?

But it was autism. We continued with full-time specialized autism Early Intervention services that were ABA-based. (ABA is applied behavior analysis, and for a two-year-old with severe autism, it is a lot of hand-over-hand repetition of forced activity.) I was in love with the therapists, and even though life was very busy, it was helpful to have people coming into the house in the beginning who knew what to do about autism. I sure didn't. I felt inadequately equipped to deal with this diagnosis or with my sudden son-stranger who appeared to view me no differently than the furniture surrounding him. He had no interest in anything except his little wooden street signs or his puzzles. Shapes. "Pre-math," the therapists called it. Great! He'll be an engineer, I thought. If he can ever talk again. Or, you know, look at people.

But I kept digging. We received a grant from Generation Rescue and took part in a three-month program, an "Intro to Biomed," if you will. A new supplement every week. Andrew's ATEC (Autism Treatment Evaluation Checklist) before we started the grant was 106. Anything higher than 104 is considered "severe" autism. At the end of the program, his ATEC was 84. We were watching our little boy come back to us, inch by little bitty inch.

We fought our homeowners' association and fenced in our back-yard so our happy little wanderer could stay safe and play outside. That was our only big, major, monster autism grievance—the scary, scary elopement tendencies. We knew how many children with autism drown each year as they wander and are drawn to water. We knew how many were "lost." We knew autism was deadly. We were so lucky that he's never been a screamer, never violent or angry. He was our happy little Buddha baby. But he was only two. We didn't know what our future would hold.

I dug deeper every day into the world of biomed and recovery. I was so angry. My little guy was improving, finally, but it didn't seem to have anything to do with Early Intervention. I was so angry—so angry that I had to find out the truth myself. Angry that I had to find out that vaccines are dangerous, that our food is poisonous, that Tylenol is really, truly poison, and that there were things I could do to help my son (and that the doctor didn't even know about them). I was so angry every single minute of every single day, it hurt to breathe. I was mad at everyone who had made the same choices I made, and at those whose children were perfectly fine (the kids who have only ADHD, allergies, and asthma . . . and have a future). I was mad at our doctor. Pharmaceutical companies. Monsanto. I was mad at everyone. Of course, I was angrier at myself than at all of them put together—for my blatant ignorance. I had unknowingly sacrificed my son on the altar of the fictitious greater good.

Our ABA therapy picked up intensity. Andrew was becoming extremely resistant. He was actually losing play skills. At the onset of therapy, he could put together any puzzle, knew dozens of shapes, and had very strong pre-math skills. Now, if we put a puzzle in front of him, he wouldn't even lift a hand. The therapists would try to do it hand over hand, and he would scream and cry real tears, yelling, "No!" over and over. He would meet my eyes across the room, with a look that said, "How could you let them do this to me?" For hours each day, my little Buddha baby, so happily encapsulated in his own world, was trying to tell me that he hated therapy. But what the hell was I supposed to do about it? All you hear about is how important ABA is for children with autism. The therapists were deeply con-flicted. He was not responding, he was even losing skills, and his behaviors were getting worse with each week. We spent many hours in dialogue about how to best help Andrew, but they were unwilling to budge from the ABA approach, and I felt like it was the wrong method for my son.

It was then I read the Thinking Moms' Revolution's book *Autism Beyond the Spectrum*. I wept as I read pieces of my own story, over, and over, and over. When I read Princess's chapter, "Son-Rise," my heart knew this would be important. A good autism mom friend (you know her as ShamROCK) knew her personally. She asked Princess to call me. The rest, as they say, is history.

My husband and I watched the videos of the therapists working with the children. With Son-Rise therapy, love and respect are the core. The therapists do not spend their time trying to make Andrew do what they want him to do. Instead, they themselves do exactly what Andrew is doing and learn to love it.

We then quit ABA. Though it has helped many children, it was not the right program for our son, and we had found something better.

Autism is a lot of things, and expensive is one of them. Doctor bills, supplements, and diet costs make our budget really tight, especially as there is no possible way for me to work. But we fundraised, and I packed my bag and headed to the Option Institute for the Son-Rise Start Up program, and my very own path to recovery.

Everything fell into place, from the funds to attend, to my mom's willingness and availability to stay with my children for the week. I started to see, really see, the good in the community that surrounded us. The friends and family who want to see Andrew succeed had faith in me and sacrificed their own time and money to help me pursue this road for him. Before I left for the Option Institute, where Son-Rise is taught, I already had a number of committed, loving, wonderful volunteers willing to give up their time to be a part of our family and this journey.

At Option, I learned everything I needed to do to set up a full-time volunteer-based Son-Rise program for Andrew in our home. I learned that my son is doing the very best he can. He is a magnificent being who has learned to do what he needs to do to deal with the overload of sensory attacks and the unpredictable world around him. I learned that my son processing things differently means he is more acutely in tune with my feelings and the environment in our home. If I am around him and I feel perfect acceptance and love, he will know, and he will respond. If I am around him and feel the deep,

deep grief I had been living, what must that feel like to him? Did he take that on? Did he think or feel for a moment that it was disappointment or sadness about something he did?

I learned that I get to choose. He stims visually for hours on his little signs, and I get to choose how that makes me feel. I can see it as socially unacceptable and try to stop him. Or I can accept who he is, knowing he is doing the best he can, and be at peace with what he's doing.

As an example: Early on, Andrew was passionately in love with road signs. My father-in-law bought him these beautiful wooden road signs, and Andrew loved them. He carried them around with him and would sit and play with them for hours on end. It was a visual stim for him, and the classic ABA approach to dealing with this is to take away the stim item. So his beloved stop signs were packed away for six months. Then we learned that he used those stop signs to deal with the world around him, that they made him feel secure and happy, and we realized we'd made a terrible, disrespectful decision by taking them away from him. When we unpacked those signs and gave them back to him, he laughed . . . belly laughed! He was delighted. He was so happy. And now that he's had a couple of months of unlimited access to them, he doesn't even use them anymore. That's the magic of Son-Rise. You don't take away what the kids need. You trust their instinct and believe that everything they do has a purpose, and you go with it.

As the week at Option passed and I learned more of these gems, my whole thought process changed, and so much healing took place in my angry little heart. What a gift to look at my son and not see a baby damaged by corporate greed who needs to be fixed. I just see my sweet boy, doing the best he can, and my intense love for him is no longer marred by the things that went wrong. I am thankful every minute of every single day. Now I know for sure that things have to change. We cannot continue on this path, as a world, with this generation of sick children and the generations to come. And I am devoted to doing my part to increase awareness of regressive autism, of GMOs, of vaccines, of Tylenol. I am devoted to encouraging the people I encounter to *think*.

Thanks to the Option Institute, I can operate from a place of peace and gratitude, not one of self-consuming bitterness. I no longer spend nights pissed off after debating vaccine-autism connections in public forums. I can choose to participate, or not. I can choose to turn off my phone. I know I cannot carry the world on my shoulders. I know I am not the only warrior out there. I can remember that not long ago, I was fighting for the other team.

Andrew now sees a DAN! doctor who is also a homeopath. She is treating his MTHFR mutations and clearing the vaccinations he reacted to. We are literally seeing our son grow by leaps and bounds every day. His ATEC score is 35. Less than a year after diagnosis, his score fell from 106 to 35. And I know in my heart that that needle will keep moving until there's no place left to move. I know it won't happen without a fight and a lot more blood, sweat, and tears, but I am prepared to move Heaven and Earth to help Andrew be his best self.

My other two children's lives are forever altered. Ava is a compassionate force, and she is Andrew's biggest cheerleader. He tells her how much he loves her with his eyes. She understands. Benjamin, in many senses, lost his twin to autism. They have not developed into playmates or best friends. In fact, Andrew spends a great deal of time avoiding Ben, because Ben is very loud and unpredictable. I spent a lot of time being angry that their twinhood was stolen from us all. But Ben intuitively knew how to do Son-Rise therapy. He instinctively knew that his best chance for eye contact was to join Andrew in Andrew's activity. He sneaks into Andrew's crib in the early morning for cuddles. He is mostly gentle and kind, and thanks to biomed and diet, completely on track developmentally now. I know that Ben and Ava will both be forces of truth in their generation. They know what happened to their brother. They know intimately what autism is, and what it does.

Some people believe that our recoveries, mine and Andrew's, will be a mirror of each other. That may be true. We've come a long, long way. We've got a lot of work to do, but we are so happy to be where we are and we are determined to choose happiness for the remainder of our journey. That, I believe, is truly the road to recovery.

We are largely supported by the community around us. I am often told that I am admired, and that people don't know how I do it. How proud I should be for working so hard to recover Andrew. How amazing it is, what we've done. And it is indeed hard work. There are days when I feel like I could scream if I have to syringe one more disgusting supplement into his mouth, or fix one more allergen-free meal. But I know the cost of giving up. I know the precious gems that reward me for my fight. The work I do now is the reason I was put on the planet. And I say, like the Kaufmans, creators of the Son-Rise program, before me said, "It was all for me."

Update

It's been two years since I sat down to write my chapter the first time. Two years ago, I believed with every fiber of my being that by now, Andrew would be recovered. That autism would be a past tense thing for us. Easy in, easy out. The right diet, the right supplements, and BAM! History. Bye, autism! Nice knowing you! Thanks for waking us up, now go on your merry way! He was not even two when he was diagnosed, so he'd be fine by kindergarten.

I was so, so, so, so wrong.

His ATEC, by and large, is a higher number than it was two years ago. This is, in part, because I was in such a *rush* to rid him of his autism that I jumped on every single bandwagon that came along. Every new popular treatment. And he's crashed, hard, twice. We've since learned that we have an underlying diagnosis of mitochondrial disease. This means, for us, that recovery is going to take longer than we had originally expected.

The first crash came after a popular treatment. He got sick, and one morning I found him blue, post-seizure. Crash two came after another very popular treatment: he got a virus, and he couldn't detox *and* fight the virus, so his body basically went into shock. He vomited for months. He lost tons of weight. He wouldn't eat anything but burnt bacon and burnt toast. After three years of keeping a gluten-, casein-, egg-, soy-, corn-free kitchen, I let the child pick out *any foods he wanted* so that he would eat. And so he ate Doritos. And Pop-Tarts. And Goldfish crackers. Meanwhile, his OAT (Organic Acids Test) for dysbiosis is clean and he is *thriving*. Color me confused. Really, really confused. Of course, we've worked our way back to healthier real foods, but it's taken a lot of time. And patience. In that app on my phone, Time Hop, every now and then I get flashbacks of myself making fun of people who feed their kids Goldfish. And I laugh. We've certainly come full circle.

I've learned so much about how very little I actually know. Here's what I do know: My son, he suffers sometimes. We've lived through a year of feces smearing. Of dirt eating. Of sudden sound sensitivity. But he suffers much less than many other children with autism. I see my friends' children screaming for hours. Seizing. Head banging.

Autism sucks a lot of the time. It stole my son's future. It stole his childhood. It stole so much happiness and carefreeness, and so many opportunities for joy. His twin doesn't even believe us that they're twins. Andrew is still nonverbal. The twins are turning five next week. We're still changing diapers. We may be for many years to come. We're sad sometimes on birthdays and on holidays, when we think about how the boys won't be in the same class at school; we are also sad that we never know what he's thinking or what he understands. It's utterly infuriating that this brain injury was preventable and that I could have stopped it. He could have had a normal life. But I also know autism steals actual lives. Children die from drowning and wandering and medical neglect every day because of autism. (Thanks to Son-Rise and the techniques I learned there, we do not live in anger or regret.)

And I also know this: this was meant to happen. Andrew was always meant to have autism. And we were always meant to raise him. And heal him. And live this experience. As he heals, the joyful milestones are even more joyful with him than they ever were with our neurotypical kids. I will always remember the first time he hung a Christmas ornament on a tree, the first time he opened a present, the first time he went on an Easter egg hunt. (All this year!) These memories are a kind of precious gift that you can't understand until you've experienced them. I know that our lives will be blessed with so many more unbelievably precious milestones and gifts *because* of autism. Not to mention I'll always treasure the people we've met along the way.

So, autism is a gift and a curse for us. All in one. But to survive the days, we focus on the gift parts.

I have also watched as *numerous* unvaccinated children have gotten a diagnosis the last two years. Yes, numerous. When I wrote my chapter the first time, I believed that autism was entirely preventable and that meant if you don't vaccinate, your baby will be just fine. Wrong again! It's the total toxic load, folks. *My* generation is so sick we cannot produce healthy babies. Vaccines are not the only evil contributing to this epidemic.

And yet vaccines are front and center in the news these days. In August 2014, there was huge excitement in our community as William Thompson stepped forward and admitted the CDC found a causal relationship between the MMR and autism and threw it in the literal trash can. Now, we're excitedly watching for the Senate hearings as the *Vaxxed* documentary drama unfolds and more people, including the co-founder of Autism Speaks, step forward and say on national TV that vaccines are not safe for everyone. These are truly exciting days we live in.

I was so overwhelmed with honor the first time I sat to write this chapter. Being part of this tremendous movement—helping the moms. Being a beacon of light for the newly diagnosed families. It was tremendous. Daily I was getting messages saying, "My friend just had a child diagnosed, will you help them?" And I'd hop on the phone or an instant messenger and tell them to go gluten- and casein-free immediately and get probiotics, and so on. Now, I rarely "take on" a new family, and when I do, I will tell them: you've got to read. I give them book titles. I point them in a direction so they can make their own choices and find their own way. I send them to Son-Rise. We've all got to walk our own path, you see. Are our kids recoverable? You bet, but I don't have the magic formula for healing. No one does, because it looks different for every family.

We had to let go of a lot of our ideas of what recovery might be for our family. We came to a place of understanding that we may be living with autism for the rest of our lives. And we accepted it. And things started to change. Just like everybody said they do when you finally accept it and let go.

2

Lone Star
Recovering Reese

I'VE HEARD IT SAID THAT PARENTING YOUR FIRST CHILD IS KIND OF like the first pancake in the batch—your attempts are throwaways because you haven't adjusted the temperature of the pan or you flipped the pancake too early or too late. When I got pregnant with my second daughter, I definitely felt that way based on all the things I'd learned (and some that needed to be unlearned) along the way during my first go at motherhood. My oldest had only breastfed for seven months, and I was determined to make it to at least a year with my second. Payton (my oldest) used disposable diapers, ate jarred purees, faced forward in a car seat at a year, and was fully vaccinated. I decided that Reese would be in cloth diapers (or none at all since I was researching elimination communication), she would benefit from baby-led weaning and extended rear-facing in her car seat, and she would be on a delayed and selective vaccination schedule.

Let me be clear—none of the parenting changes were influenced by autism. Autism wasn't on my radar any more than Pendred syndrome, encephalopathy, chronic diarrhea, seizures, or mitochondrial dysfunction were. My decisions were only based on some sort of ideal I had at the time—the pursuit of crunchiness, I suppose. Autism didn't creep onto my screen until Reese was a toddler.

Put simply, I was going to do better for Reese (and Payton) by being healthier and more "natural." But I now know that there is a huge divide between better and best. Being better, doing better, feeding better, and treating better are all just statements of comparison with actions that are worse. I could say I'm eating healthier if I choose Chick-Fil-A over McDonald's and, technically, I might be correct, but I'm certainly not eating the healthiest diet I can. I learned these lessons the hard way when Reese turned one.

Disclaimer: I recount these incidents as though I was fully cognizant of them at the time; I wasn't. My hindsight is 20/20, so I've had to piece together events through photos, emails, and rough recollection. Until autism walked into our home uninvited, I wasn't a note-taker. I have no baby books for any of my kids. Now, I have medical record binders and day planners full of notes about what's been eaten, what supplements were taken, what the mood of the day was.

On Friday, January 26, 2012, the day before Reese's first birthday, she had her one-year well-child checkup. Her doctor, whom I adored, and I had agreed upon a staggered and selective immunization schedule. On that date, she was in need of her Hib shot. I dutifully complied with the imposed rules. Two days later, as friends and family members gathered to celebrate her birthday, she seemed out-of-sorts. She sat quietly on her grandfather's lap, spending the majority of the party hugging a balloon. We don't have a single photo of her smiling that day.

From that date forward, it was one mysterious medical event after another. Unexplained fevers and rhinitis occurred in February. March started with her no longer responding to her name, followed by odd marks presenting on the front of her feet. Her doctor was perplexed by them because the marks didn't match any kind of common rash or dermatological reaction to chemicals, nor were they the result of trauma or intense heat. He mentioned the possibility of an autoimmune connection, but the marks eventually faded and disappeared completely after a month, so we didn't discuss a potential systemic cause any further.

Soon after, she experienced what appeared to be a gnarly diaper rash. Being the healthier, crunchier, better mama, I immediately busted out the coconut oil and slathered it on along with cow's milk yogurt applied directly to the area. Plus, she enjoyed frequent diaper-free time while we tried to start potty training. But the rash worsened tenfold and spread. She began bleeding and crying out in pain. Her doctor diagnosed it as yeast and then, a couple of weeks later, he surmised that it had become staph. But prescription ointments didn't touch it, nor did a broad-spectrum antibiotic. And then, just like the marks before it, the rash went away.

By May, I had decided to do a hearing test as it was becoming obvious that my daughter wasn't attending to peripheral noise. In fact, one morning her sister came bounding down the stairs shouting: "Good morning, Reese!" Reese didn't notice Payton until she was directly in her line of sight. The ENT discovered fluid so thick that her ear drums couldn't move, yet she had never had an ear infection. Even though she had just finished a course of strong antibiotics, and the doctor had determined that the fluid was uninfected, he wanted her to take more antibiotics along with steroids. I reluctantly agreed to the steroids, but refused the antibiotics. After three days on her meds, I found her to be aggressive and violent, plus she had vomited at least once, so we ceased that course of treatment.

I did some research and decided to have her seen twice a week by a chiropractor and to administer mullein garlic oil drops at home as a more natural way of treating her ears. When we went to the follow-up at the ENT's office and I proudly told him how we chose to treat her ears, he quipped, "I'm sure we will have to put in some tubes." Then he peeked in her ears and found they were clear and her hearing had been restored. He backpedaled a bit, but insisted that while the chiropractor didn't do any harm, it probably wasn't what worked.

That summer, her diaper rash returned, looking somewhat different than before. A dermatologist diagnosed her with Jacquet's dermatitis, a rare skin disorder brought on by prolonged exposure to moisture. She recommended using disposable diapers and declined to do any further testing, though Reese's PCP had referred us for that purpose. I complied with the recommendation and boxed up all the cloth diapers.

Not long after, Reese had her highest fever to date—over 104 degrees. She seemed perfectly fine otherwise, just a little tired. She drifted into a quiet sleep on my chest (I enjoyed her snuggles), and I assumed she would sleep it off and wake up cooler and happier. About twenty minutes into her nap, however, her body jerked suddenly. Though I noticed it, I wrote it off as just dreamy movements. Then another jerk, and another. I rushed her to urgent care and was told to give her Tylenol for the fever. Confused, I asked the doctor if that would just prolong it and even increase the risk of the fever spiking back up and causing another seizure. He stated, rather frankly, "Yes, but if she's hot, she's uncomfortable, and you want to make her *feel* better."

Throughout all this time, Reese was a totally different girl than she had been as an infant. Her funny personality was gone. The words she had started using around eleven months were lost, and she expressed little interest in learning new words. She threw tantrums frequently, seemingly without provocation. And she stopped accepting affection; hugs and kisses had to be on her terms and when she prompted them. All of these doctors had seen her, but we had no answers. I was happily given prescriptions, but no solutions. The light bulb went off as I left urgent care. What am I doing to myself and what am I doing to her? Why?

From then on, I was noting behaviors and symptoms—the staring spells, the hand-flapping, the toe walking, the sensory-seeking, the lack of awareness of danger or her surroundings in general, poop play, spinning, humming, fingers in the eyes, aggressive outbursts, violence, parallel play at preschool, red spots around her mouth, dark circles under her eyes, uncontrollable bowels. To this day, I come across misplaced pieces of paper with my scribbled notes and find lists I wrote on my phone.

The mountain of evidence was growing taller and taller each day, yet her Early Intervention therapists who had started coming to the home seemed unconcerned. Twice a week they came and paid no mind to the way Reese regarded them as strangers every time. I had to push for an M-CHAT, which I was told she "failed." (The M-CHAT—Modified Checklist for Autism in Toddlers—is a developmental screening tool designed to identify children who may need a more thorough autism evaluation.)

So began another long series of specialist visits, a series that has yet to conclude. Neurologist, ENT, audiologist, allergist, gastroenterologist, geneticist, endocrinologist, DAN! (Defeat Autism Now!) doctor, MAPS (Medical Academy of Pediatric Special Needs) doctor, naturopath, speech, and occupational therapists. By now, though, I had learned my lessons: Do not take "no" or "I don't know" for an answer. Do not accept defeat. Do not fill prescriptions unless there is imminent danger in not doing so. Do not do anything but the best for her. Do not ignore my gut. Do not ignore my child.

As I look back and add up all the pieces in this awful equation, I see dominoes toppling over. The immediate brain fog—encephalopathy. The odd marks—immune system overload. The diaper rashes—goat milk intolerance and gluten sensitivity causing dermatitis herpetiformis. The glue ear, red spots, dark circles—more immune system overload. The staring spells—more seizures. The explosive poops—leaky gut, inflammation, mitochondrial dysfunction. The odd behaviors—manifestations and symptoms of larger systemic problems that all add up to an autism diagnosis.

Autism is now my life. It is my job. I'm like a clean-up crew after a natural disaster, or better yet, a crime scene investigator. All of the pieces need to be meticulously and patiently scrutinized and researched if I am to find a solution and recover my daughter.

Through tireless work I am doing just that—recovering Reese. I still see all of those mainstream specialists; if you're on a tight budget with bad insurance, it's the only way to get tests done without breaking the bank. But I take their advice with a huge boulder of salt, then have her MAPS doc, her GI specialist, and her local ND review it all. And although I trust them more than other practitioners because of their deeper knowledge of children with developmental disorders, I still make decisions based on my gut and my child. If it weren't for those standards I have set for myself and her treatment, I would not have discovered her genetic hearing loss, or her fecal impactions, or her night seizures. I push, I fight, and for good reason.

She has started coming back to us. Her eye contact is strong, her empathy improving. She finally recognizes herself in photos, and loves to be imaginative in her play. She drew a stick figure the other day and has started calling her sister "bubba" again! Reese is an amazing, brave, and strong little girl. She has endured so much in such a short time, and we aren't even a quarter of the way there. Because of her, I am now the best mom I can be, and I'm no longer willing to settle for just "better."

3

Monarch

From Lost and Hopeless to Healing and Action

"I never thought your life would turn out this way," my mom said to me in a whisper with a voice crack that exposed her pain and undermined her attempt to keep her composure. Her efforts were too late, as I had noted her eyes rimming red.

Her words hit me like a truck. We were separated from the rest of the family and near the couch during Thanksgiving dinner at my house. I sat with my parents and husband at the dining room table, which was being bombarded by little fingers belonging to my four-year-old twins, who reached from behind chairs, grabbed at plates, and scooped little fistfuls of food only to smell it and drop it to the floor, smear it on the wall, or rub it into the carpet.

The twins kept the dinner lively with meltdowns, shrieks, wails, outbursts of aggression, and throwing of toys. As the topic of conversation was kept light to balance the tension and obvious abnormal circumstances of the meal, suddenly her words, meaningful, sorrowful, and heavy, felt like a gash, an old wound opened in my flesh.

Her simple statement broke through my façade, and I felt my life exposed. "This way" was all that was needed to be said between the two of us for her meaning to be perfectly clear. The loss, the constant struggle, challenges, exhaustion, financial devastation, frequent medical appointments, and fight against multiple agencies and entities that had become my norm were all brought to the surface by her innocent admission. My mother never thought my life would turn out this way. She never thought I would have children with autism—two of them.

How could I be surprised by these words as we were surrounded by the noise, the wails, the children's refusal to sit, and the throwing of toys swirling around us? Despite my days of cleaning, toys covered the floor in rooms with torn furniture, carpets ruined by urine, feces, vomit, spit-up supplements, and numerous foods that were refused and hurled across the room. The old saying goes, "If these walls could talk . . ." My walls did talk, and they revealed my life inside them to all. My walls held back no secrets and hid nothing. They spoke volumes. Once pristine, the walls were now covered in markers, pens, holes, cracks, chipped paint, large patches of drywall ripped away from toys being flung against them, and hundreds of dents due to repeated hits with a toy. Not one wall was without a battle scar.

I was in one of my moments where I had to turn down the chaos, the crying, the screaming, and the throwing of objects past me and focus instead on what to do next. Should I calm four-year-old Nathan, who was wailing demands that none of his toys be moved from their obsessively positioned places, or pull off the coffee table Nathan's twin brother, William, who was screaming and shrieking while punching himself in the head? The chaos escalated as Willy ruined Nathan's carefully laid out pattern, causing Nathan to disintegrate into shrieks of panic, obsessive word repetition, and intense biting of his forearm. Willy attempted to hit and shove anyone in his personal space to quiet the unwanted noise. He began his own screaming, slamming his head with his fists and clawing at his neck with his fingernails. Nathan screeched again and again, "He broke it! He broke it! Bring it back!"

The words, while painful, loud, and angry, were still pure music and joy to me. Thank God for Nathan's words. Although not conversational, he was able to express his frustration through his tears and screaming—he wanted control and the small order he had found in his spinning and unsteady world was now demolished. Willy was rendered with no way to express his anger, sadness, internal chaos, continual abdominal pain, and his feelings of being overwhelmed in his surroundings, except to explode into aggression and screaming. He hung his head, sitting still but with his body shaking and heaving with silent sobs. No feeling is more complicated and painful than watching the people you love the most be controlled by pain inflicted by the thing you hate the most. Looking at my sons, I simultaneously see the most beautiful part of my life and the most painful.

In addition to their explosive and atypical behaviors, the twins were wrought with medical challenges, which our pediatrician brushed off as unimportant. The twins were constantly afflicted with diarrhea, only occasionally broken by constipation. Their stools were liquid, pale, or green, and they caused horrible rashes. Eating was a challenge as they fought every feeding and often threw up after. They had severe gastric reflux, to the point of crying for hours after a feeding, which the pediatrician stated was simply normal for preemies. Since birth, they were incredibly poor sleepers. They never slept more than an hour and a half at a time and seemed agitated in their sleep as they kicked and groaned. Willy constantly grimaced as if in pain, and never, ever stopped kicking his feet. Both had hundreds of little white bumps all over their arms, back, and chest, and odd rashes came and went. They were in a constant state of irritation and agitation as if the whole world, every touch and sound, was painful to them.

I frequently mentioned these concerns to their pediatrician, who said it was simply "SPS": Stupid Preemie Stuff. However, as the boys grew, these problems only got worse. The sleep, the diarrhea, the rashes, the food refusal, the kicking, and the crying continued without abatement and without understanding.

My heart ached to look at them, and yet I felt a certain hope. Having a child with autism means always searching for the hope and continuing to move forward. You must diligently treat the bodily injuries that are causing the behaviors and use even an emotionally charged moment like this to step back objectively to determine and monitor the effectiveness of the path you're on to heal them.

Healing and improvements, although slow and wrought with setbacks, had occurred in my sons due to continued treatments and diet. Nathan was expressing his frustration, and Willy was calming himself. We had come so far, and yet we had a long journey ahead of us.

I continued to watch Willy and refocused on my mother, who was right by my side attempting to calm the storm, one of many that day. Her comment had now fully taken possession of my thoughts. I analyzed her statement and wondered what response she was seeking. I had no answer. How had my life turned out? The statement was one of pity and empathy, almost an apology. She meant well. I inhaled, now feeling my eyes begin to sting, and remained silent so as not to reveal my own cracked voice. The words were ambiguous to a degree. "*This way.*" My mother never thought my life would turn out "this way." What was the "way" in her comment? The diagnosis of autism in my twin boys, one profound and severe and the other moderate, was the obvious answer, but the autism diagnosis was just a label.

In what "way" had autism stolen my family's normalcy, its sense of safety and protection, its place in society, its ability to engage in the average events of day-to-day living? Was it having four-year-olds in diapers? My sons' bodies, internal systems, and organs injured and overloaded with toxins? Willy's nonverbal state except for the almost constant screaming? Nathan on the verge of an uncontrollable meltdown at the most innocuous events? The financial ruin of my family? The loss of friends and family as the twins grew and the autism became more obvious, more undeniable? The necessity for me to become a twenty-four-hour caregiver? The way we stood out in public like the neon lights of Vegas as the boys got older and their lack of language and infantile behavior became more pronounced? No words or narratives are sufficient to accurately and completely describe the life of caring for a child with autism. Life with autism is a personal experience and challenge for every family; it is constantly changing and evolving.

I was being naïve and thoughtless. Her statement was sincere and her disbelief understandable. In fact, if she had not been shocked that I became a mother of twins with autism, it would be unusual. Of course my mother was stunned by the events that unfolded in my life. None of this was supposed to happen. When she raised me, autism was not part of the national vocabulary, not even a blip on the radar. Autism was not discussed or feared; it was not even part of the American consciousness. Our family's journey and familiarity with autism began before I was even born and had not yet revealed itself for its true nature.

Autism entered my mother's sphere of awareness at a time when autism was rare—1 case in 10,000 children. But long before autism became part of the national fabric and a medical and cultural phenomenon, it had already touched our lives and shaped my mother's thinking and perception of autism. She had understood autism as a mysterious psychiatric condition that surely would never touch her life, let alone having two grandsons struggle with the condition. However, even then, as I was a child of the 1970s and teenager of the 1980s, the stage was being set and the pieces put into place for the most wide-sweeping epidemic of our modern age.

We entered an age of tremendously increasing toxicity in our environment, and those toxins were directly entering our bodies. The pharmaceutical companies were competing in a vaccine race to create the first vaccine for any given disease to add to the childhood vaccine schedule. The FDA and CDC, with their links to Congressional politicians whose campaigns are largely financed by pharmaceutical companies, were poised and ready to support these national advancements in healthcare. Toxins from new products meant to make our lives easier and more efficient were introduced into our environment at an alarming rate, and advancements in agriculture and food production were being widely studied and utilized (such as increased pesticides, additives, and preservatives). We were so woefully unaware, so painfully ignorant to the storm coming to crush our world along with that of hundreds of thousands of other families. My mom had come miles from her 1970s perception of autism. She was the first to meet our enemy.

The 1960s and 1970s were a time of experimentation, civil unrest, and the idea that the individual could change the world. During this turbulent but exciting climate, Vivienne, a young graduate student studying child psychology and development at the University of Illinois, and also my future mother, stood with her fellow classmates outside the Adler Zone, the university's psychiatric unit. The professor, having talked up this outing in the prior class, had left the students with hopes of something rare and exotic behind the door. The year was 1969, and it seemed at the time that the study of psychiatry had already firmly defined most deviations of the brain, behavior, and thought. What could be so new, rare, and unexplored that these students, lacking in experience and having not yet earned their advanced degree, would be permitted to examine and observe it? Before opening the door, the professor said something that haunts me, the daughter of the young and eager graduate student, even now in moments of exhaustion and frustration. He spoke with intent and the rambunctious group became quiet at his words: "You are extremely lucky to observe this subject. I promise you, no matter how far you go and despite how long you pursue your careers in psychology, you will never witness this again. Never." The excitement quieted to a hush. The door opened to reveal a fourteen-year-old boy. His diagnosis: autism.

My mother's assignment was to use basic ABA (applied behavior analysis) to modify his behaviors. The boy's mother was always present during the sessions. My mother recalls often thinking how his mother must have felt so isolated, having no answers, knowing no others with a child suffering with the same condition. Little did she know how intimate she would become with the thoughts, fears, and hopes of another mother with a child with autism.

Since my mother's first introduction to autism decades ago, autism has become a national epidemic and crisis. The year my sons were diagnosed, 2009, the US autism rates were released by the CDC: an astonishing 1 in 250. I was devastated and angry. All these injuries could have been prevented. As I write this, the latest number released by the CDC is 1 in 50 school-aged children. These numbers will continue to rise as our children are assaulted with ever-increasing toxins while a majority of society remains complacent. However, there is a whisper, a ripple, even a current, of change in the climate. Mothers and fathers are learning the truth and sharing their stories. More doctors and specialists are questioning how and why our children are becoming sicker with each generation.

Forty years after my mother provided ABA to the boy with the extremely rare condition known as autism, I frantically called her on a Wednesday night in July 2009 to hysterically proclaim that my seventeen-month-old twin sons, William and Nathan, had autism. She laughed. Trying to calm me, she reminded me of my exhaustion, lack of sleep, and tendency to worry excessively about the twins, and she told me to simply relax. Everything would be fine. After all, she had seen them only ten days earlier. Their behavior was typical, playful, curious, and affectionate. She would know, having a Master's degree in Child Development and Psychology. She could not understand that the unfolding of events in a mere ten days changed my life, my sons' lives, and my family's lives forever.

Five days before my desperate call, my typical twin boys had received their MMR shots and three other vaccinations. The nurses reminded us to administer Tylenol before they went to bed to reduce soreness. By that evening, the Tylenol seemed like a good idea as both were hot and sweaty with fever. They were listless and barely resisted the Tylenol syringe as they typically did. The next day, as if their skin or bodies were being irritated, the boys were agitated with fever and unable to sit still or rest. They were not interested in their favorite toys and activities. That evening, as I sang to Willy and held him in my arms, he stared, almost without blinking, at his nightlight turtle. As I blocked his line of vision with my face, he would simply move his head, his gaze glued to the light. He persisted in fixating on the turtle as I headed for the door, and for first time ever he did not cry when I left the room. He did not even notice. Nathan, slick with sweat and pink from fever, was already asleep when I entered his room. His face was not the relaxed and slackened face of a slumbering toddler—it was tight and crunched. He tossed and kicked all through the night. He woke often and rambled gibberish to the walls as he ignored me and my gentle kisses. He got out of bed in the morning glassy-eyed and dazed; his usually bright eyes were distant and bland.

As their fever and "sickness" passed, something greater and more profound had taken hold. They seemed changed, different, distant, even younger and more infantile. They lost interest in toys, began flapping their arms, toe walking, and licking and mouthing every surface including the floor and walls. Their personalities, previously so bright, big, and luminous, became flat, lifeless, expressionless, and irritable. Their language was gone, their sense of wonder at new things transformed from exploration to staring at fans; they were fascinated by anything with repetitive motion or sound. I knew instantly and completely that something immense, something affecting their whole body and biology, had changed. They had not simply developed unusual tendencies or lost a few new behaviors; they were different children. I stayed up night after night with my computer looking up their symptoms, and every search returned the same result: autism.

We immediately arranged a team diagnostic testing of our sons. Six months was the average wait time for the appointment.

I found myself falling down a dark black hole where no air, no life, no light could penetrate the deep darkness that had swallowed me. I did not know it then, but the person I had been, the foundation upon which I based my life, was about to disintegrate, and I would now move forward with no ground beneath my feet. But I proceeded with eyes wide open where once they had been unknowingly closed. Ignorance is bliss, and my own Eden had just been set on fire. The institutions I trusted, the moral code I believed we as a community of humanity upheld, the safety measures and protections created and enforced by my government, the belief that modern medicine and the healthcare system existed to ensure my well-being and protect the food that nourished me, and the very basis of my intricate understanding of the world all no longer existed—and never really had existed. My prior life—my prior *self*—was dead.

I felt lost, alone, and in a deep despair that left me deflated and disoriented. The world seemed colorless. I felt my family played no part in this world, had no role in society. Everything was a reminder of our differences. Every child on the playground, every picture on Facebook of a child proudly holding their honor roll certificate, every television show and commercial with precocious and clever kids outwitting their parents and neatly navigating their way through the world were all reminders of what my sons could not be, a reminder of all their potential that was lost.

In the very early stages, despite my despair, I could not wait to begin treatment, any treatment. I needed movement, regardless of direction. My sons were different, faded, and seemed ill. I was losing myself, yet I continued to fight for my sons. However, because I neglected to take care of myself and manage my devastation, my decisions for my sons' treatment and care were affected. I was moving too fast with no direction or path. I wanted to try everything and try it now. If I read something worked for someone on Facebook or heard it in a support group, I chased it without reason. Any new treatment or the latest supplement became my next pursuit in healing my sons, but I did so without actually understanding their underlying medical conditions. I was utterly destroyed and incapable of seeing the bigger picture in terms of their treatment. The overall treatment of the complex integration and the synthesis of the body's processes and systems were not part of my rationale. I wanted to run the sprint, not the marathon. I was lost and so was the path to their healing.

I started using biomedical treatments and ABA therapy in the home when the twins were eighteen months, but I knew recovery was not promised. Despite moving forward with treatments, I was still blind and weighted down with grief and the need for immediate and immense progress. Without that ironclad promise of defeating autism, I felt as though I had no ground beneath my feet. I wanted a guarantee. I was chasing random treatments without proper research or guidance in my decisions. I found myself and my sons spinning in circles, and progress was slow. I couldn't sit on my hands and do nothing and wait six months for these appointments to tell me what I already knew. I took to the Internet for answers.

From day one, I accepted the challenge to take on autism rather than simply accept it as an untreatable condition. Every free moment I had, I researched and read. I absorbed as much information as I could. I joined support groups. Initially, my research was random and rushed, leading to treatments based on popularity rather than my sons' unique medical injuries. Seeing no progress, I quickly began to approach my research in a more methodical way and used the data and labs from my MAPS doctor to decide our path. (MAPS doctors are leaders in the medical community who believe in treating the biological and medical comorbidities of children with autism in order to heal and recover them, rather than simply trying to modify the children's behaviors. MAPS doctors operate on the foundation that autism is medical and therefore treatable through medical interventions.) The number of books, studies, and treatment options was overwhelming. In my mind, I divided the treatments into two approaches.

The first theory was that autism was a set of behaviors that could be shaped and controlled with therapies and reinforcers. I ordered book after book about engaging autism, games to play, and behaviorism. Every word was a painful swallow of a drink I did not want to imbibe. All the "answers" were advice for how to manage autism, to contain it and control it. I wanted it gone. I wanted to cure it. I wanted my babies back and nothing less. They were ill.

In my mind, shaping their behavior alone did not resolve how one day a bright-eyed curious child became a sick, sullen, isolated, shrieking ball of pain, bumps, rashes, diarrhea, constipation, inability to sleep, and refusal to eat all but three foods. I did not know the extent or nature of their injuries, but I knew my twins needed more than stacking blocks and matching pictures.

As I rapidly refined my research and understanding of my sons' injuries and learned to interpret their labs, I found myself drawn to the second school of thought, which argued that autism is a medical condition often brought on by injury or trauma to the infant or child through toxins—vaccines often being the biggest culprit— entering their bodies and wreaking havoc on the delicate balance of their various organs, biological systems, and even cells. We are bombarded with toxins every day, in our foods through GMOs and pesticides, our home cleansers, fertilizers, and unnecessary medications. I would not accept living this way. I had chosen our path. I was going to treat my sons' injuries, heal their guts and inflamed immune systems, take control of their diets, and supplement their nutrient-deficient bodies.

As we waited for the months to pass to be given an "official" diagnosis from a team of experts who would examine the boys' behaviors to determine their condition, I had already taken them to see a MAPS doctor, run a panel of tests, completed a stool testing, begun a gluten-free, casein-free, and soy-free diet, become an involved member of a biomedical information and support group, and had met other mothers on this path. I had listened to their stories of treatments and healing approaches, such as HBOT, chelation, various diets for healing the gut, viral treatments, homeopathic treatments, herbal remedies, and countless other treatments.

I found a well-respected and highly regarded MAPS doctor, Dr. Anju Usman, and was amazed to learn she was a local doctor. She ordered various preliminary tests, the results of which shocked me and at the same time made perfect sense. The Comprehensive Stool Analysis revealed their guts were full of yeast, their count literally surpassed the top of the chart. A Urine Toxic Metals Test showed that their metals, particularly aluminum and mercury, were past normal limits. Their viral counts were out of control (as we learned from a Viral Load Test). Nathan's measles and rubella titers were so high that he tested positive for both diseases, and we were actually contacted by our state's Department of Health and had to get a note from the pediatrician in order for him to return to school.

As we advanced into testing, the twins also underwent a DNA Microarray Analysis genetic test that determined that both of them suffered from mitochondrial dysfunction; Willy also had lactic acidosis. The mito result demonstrated that their cells were not functioning properly. I will not catalog all of their ailments and disturbing test results, but the tests were clear and absolute: my children were sick. Test after test revealed disturbing results and countless injuries and traumas.

I learned how my taking a strong antibiotic a month before labor had disturbed my sons' delicate gut flora. The gut, being the center of the immune system, once compromised creates infants and children with weak immune systems and inflammation. My sons' guts had formed holes, allowing toxins to easily pass through to their bloodstream and through the blood–brain barrier, causing neurological injury. After delivery, I remained in the hospital for five days for a severe infection with three IVs pumping me full of what the nurses assured me were the three strongest antibiotics they had. I was breast-feeding. I was destroying their guts; I was causing inflammation, and their immune systems were being challenged and taxed.

The boys had their first pediatric gastroenterologist appointment at four weeks. Over the next year, they would see three more GI specialists with no results. Because of reflux, they screamed and cried as they ate. They were endlessly restless, irritable, and inconsolable. They had already experienced their first injury prior to birth, and their bodies were weak, inflamed, and immune-compromised when they received their fifteen-month vaccines. Once the vaccines entered their weakened bodies, the real damage began, and they began to fade from me.

The more I learned about autism as a medical condition, the more hope swelled up inside me. Medical conditions can be and are treated. I sensed that even though the undertaking was enormous and extremely complicated, with the information and support of the autism community and treatments from the handful of doctors that recognized autism for its medical nature, I could make sure autism was not in control of my life. Autism could be managed and treated. We began treating our sons with guarded enthusiasm, and I had to learn to follow their lead by watching their behavior and reactions to treatment. I also had to understand that I was the one in control, not autism. I saw gains, stagnation, and glimpses of hope. I realized that a promise of recovery was not what I needed to create a new identity to navigate this world.

Instead, I needed to be empowered. Empowered with knowledge that treatments were available and that I could guide my sons' healing. Empowered to understand that autism is not a mysterious condition and lifelong sentence, but rather a medical condition. Empowered that the knowledge and information to heal my sons were out there—I simply had to seek it out. The more I read and researched, and the more knowledge I gained, the more empowered

I became. Autism had been in control of my direction and perceptions; now *I* was. I knew autism was fightable. I could move forward in hope and knowledge rather than stagnate in fear and misunderstanding. As I began to see my sons peek through their shells, I began to withdraw from mine.

Autism was no longer a monster that had a hold on my sons. I was in charge of my sons' recovery and therefore I was in charge of the "autism." We have used multiple biomedical approaches. Some have yielded great advancement, and some have had little effect. For me, climbing out of the darkness and into the light and becoming a real fighter was not always about winning, but rather about the awareness that I controlled the path. I did not have to be at the mercy of endless diarrhea and bowel issues, viruses, inflammation, immune compromise, and mitochondrial dysfunction. I realized that I had endless resources of books, studies, research, other caregiver's stories, and MAPS doctors to guide my decisions. I. Could. Think. I am a Thinker.

Thinking is empowering. Thinking puts you in charge of your child's recovery, of their treatments and path. Thinking shrinks autism down from a stomping and uncontrollable monster consuming your life and dominating your fears, your pain, and your dread of the future. You can slay the monster and reduce it to a medical problem that can be revealed through labs, stool cultures, and other testing. Thinking means you understand that autism is avoidable and treatable—recovery is possible. Thinking does not guarantee recovery but guides you and your next step to fight autism. Even when autism seems to have its claws deep in your child, never forget you are in charge. Even when your child is banging their head against the wall, or smearing feces on the carpet, or melting down right in front of you, you are in charge. You have the power to examine and determine the underlying reasons and attack them with might, determination, and science-based treatments. This revelation saved me, pulling me out of isolation, despair, and my belief that our future was set and bleak.

I went through a transformation, a rebirth, a chrysalis period where I learned the causes of autism, that autism is an injury, not a set of behaviors, and that autism is treatable. I carved the path using my children's behaviors and medical tests. I researched endlessly, devoured books about various treatments to heal the body, and grew wings to fly. Now, like a butterfly soaring high in the air, I could look down and see it all: the path, the paradise in the distance, and the hope of a better future. I recognized that I didn't need the ground beneath my feet and the stability that I had believed a guarantee of recovery would provide me. Letting go of your loss and your need for a promise that every treatment is the right one and that recovery is around the corner frees you of your grief and your need to hold onto what should have been. This allows you to focus on treatment and finding the right path. You will make mistakes. You will spend time, money, and energy on treatments that don't work for your child, but these are not failures. These are just road blocks showing you another direction. Keep moving forward.

Knowledge is Power. Ignorance is Bliss. One may choose to live in blind happiness, or one may choose to live an informed and purposeful life, but at a cost. Along with knowledge, one must face and internalize harsh truths about our society and corruption in our government, our corporations, and our medical community that keep our children sick. I hate autism. I hate what it has done to my sons, my daughter, and my family. If autism had not entered my life, I would probably be living my typical American life with my three kids, a career, two cars in the garage, and a nice, modest home. However, I would also be drinking diet sodas, eating pesticide-laden foods and processed "foods" with toxic GMOs instead of nutrition. I would be vaccinating, getting flu shots, and filling my body with neurotoxins and poisons that attack the immune system, the gut, and the brain, and cause havoc in my body so deep and profound that it has the power to injure and change the function and health of my cells. I would also be doing this to my family.

Autism gave me the power of sight. Autism first broke me and then sent me on a journey for answers that changed me and my entire perspective and understanding of society, government, medicine, corporations, and science. The more I learned, the stronger I became. I gave up crawling on the ground and eating the crumbs dropped down to me from the powers above. I grew wings and soared above the lies and corruption to a state of truth and empowerment. We—the mothers, fathers, and caregivers of injured children carrying the "autism" label—are the holders of the truth, which gives us tremendous power. We have an enormous responsibility to spread this truth, to never allow it to be buried or covered, and to continue to fight for our children.

Our mission is to spread this truth to every community, every parent, and every individual. Change begins by sweeping away old dogmas and lies told by corporations, agencies, and the government. Our biggest weapon against their forced propaganda and cover-up attempts: our stories. We spread the truth by telling our stories of what happened to our children, how they became sick, and how we are healing them. Our stories will shed light on the darkness and pull others out of the darkness of ignorance, even at the cost of their false bliss. Our stories will enlighten the world and change society's perspective, shake people out of complacency, and allow them to ask questions and initiate their own research. The truth will set you free, and our stories are our truth. We will change the world perspective if we are not afraid to use our voices and share. Hundreds of thousands of us have a story to tell. This one is mine.

4

Hoppy
There Is a Voice That Doesn't Use Words. Listen.

OVER TWO YEARS AGO, I WAS SITTING IN THE BASEMENT WITH my twenty-one-month-old son Jack, my husband, and Jack's developmental therapist. My five-week-old baby boy was asleep upstairs. Jack had just finished his third weekly therapy session and had run off to throw toys on the floor, as he did very often back then. Since we had not yet had a real conversation about what was going on with him, I decided to bring up autism with his therapist.

I knew the answer already, but having my fears confirmed by an expert broke my heart into a million pieces. She sat with us patiently, giving us little pieces of hope as she described seeing other kids improve after the elimination of dairy and gluten from their diet. She also mentioned Jenny McCarthy's book, which I immediately discounted ("Isn't she, like, anti-vaccine?"). Still, I read the book when she brought it to me the next week. I was desperate. I am so grateful to this day that our therapist was open-minded enough to put me on the right path.

The beginning of my story is not so different from that of most mothers of special children. My son was born vulnerable. He had lots of stress, was sick a lot, and received all of the recommended vaccinations. At around eighteen months, we realized that something was wrong because he wasn't talking and barely looked at us anymore. He entered our state's Early Intervention program and started speech, occupational, and developmental therapy. That first day his therapist mentioned "autism" to us, I thought my life was over. I felt like I didn't know this beautiful boy at all anymore, and maybe I never had. It seemed like the end of a dream. But in reality, it was just the beginning of a better life for all of us.

My son has been under stress his whole life, beginning with his conception. A year before Jack was born, our first baby was stillborn at thirty-two weeks. It was unexpected, unexplained, and unbelievably devastating to my husband and me. We decided to move forward quickly to try to ease the pain, and conceived Jack about five months after losing her.

It was a wonderfully uneventful pregnancy, but it was very stressful. I constantly worried that it would happen again. I had over twenty ultrasounds to monitor my son and ensure that all was well. My OB and high-risk specialist agreed that I should be induced at thirty-seven weeks. I was grateful for all of the interventions and just wanted him out and alive. I had no idea what I was setting him up for.

My induction lasted for three days. I was given drugs to dilate my cervix, then massive amounts of Pitocin to push him out. He needed vacuum extraction after I pushed for two hours and was too exhausted from the induction process to keep going. Back then, I was unaware of the huge amount of stress I was putting my baby under by forcing him out early.

He was a beautiful baby, just shy of seven pounds at birth. He had a ton of dark hair and big dark eyes. But he was a tired baby. He could not stay awake long enough to nurse. He had terrible jaundice that required an overnight hospital stay when he was just three days old. I was instructed to give him formula or else he would never be able to excrete the bilirubin. I did as I was told.

The first several weeks of his brand new life were, again, stressful. He cried a lot. He would curl up as though his tummy was just killing him. He would sleep only while moving, so he spent a lot of time in the swing, and we took a lot of car rides. I asked questions about dairy allergies, reflux, and gas. Our pediatrician brushed me off, saying that there was no research to support any of my ideas. I cut out dairy from my diet anyway, and it seemed to help. We found a new pediatrician.

Then, of course, there were the shots. He got them all. Twenty-nine different vaccinations between birth and eighteen months of age. My son did not have an obvious regression after his vaccines. He was, however, constantly sick. He had colds, RSV (respiratory syncytial virus), two ear infections, and a sinus infection before he was nine months old. He was in daycare, and everyone told me this was to be expected, that it was building up his immune system. He never slept during the day; he was so stressed by the noise and commotion. They said he was a happy baby, which made me feel better, but now I know he was just in his own world. He spent a lot of time in the jumper as he got bigger—he would jump all day if we let him, trying desperately to organize his body and get the input that he needed.

I wish I'd never put him there—leaving my brand new baby, my most precious little person, alone with strangers for over eight hours a day at such a young and vulnerable age was the first of many times that I did not listen to my inner voice. I often wonder if he felt abandoned or scared during those long days, if that caused him to withdraw into himself a bit more each day. Later, during the first year of his Heilkunst treatment, we cleared the trauma of daycare from his timeline. That week, as we drove by the daycare building on the way to his preschool, I was reminded of that sad feeling I used to have when I left him there. Just then, a little voice from my backseat said softly, "Mommy sad, baby sad." I almost ran off the road because

I was so surprised—my nonverbal three-year-old had not only read my mind, but also seemed to be recalling both of our feelings from those days. I still almost don't believe it happened, but I know it did.

When he was nine months old, my mom retired and started watching him full time. He seemed to catch up then. He started crawling, rolling over, and babbling a little, and the sickness faded. He was still a cranky little guy, though; he was very particular about his routines, would not sleep without being held, and cried a lot. He spent a lot of time jumping, playing with toys that lit up and played music, and watching TV—the only things that seemed to calm him.

I stopped breast-feeding when he was thirteen months old and I was pregnant again. After that, he steadily lost touch with his world—his eye contact and engagement fading day by day—and his developmental progress had slowed to a halt by the time he was eighteen months.

I've never been able to pinpoint the moment, or day, or week that it happened. I've looked at photos, watched videos, and searched my brain for memories of his eye contact, his engagement, his development. Where did it all go wrong? I believe now that it was happening all along, and started even before birth. Gradually, life became too much for him, and he faded away into his own world of repetitive play and sensory seeking behaviors.

I try not to dwell on the diagnosis or my feelings about the causes of my son's condition. The guilt still gets to me at times. I vividly remember completely ignoring my own gut instincts about many things—the induction, formula supplements, daycare, so very many shots—but back then I didn't trust myself. I went with the flow. All of my friends did what I was doing, and their kids seemed perfectly fine. It was very difficult to accept that my decisions had caused so much trauma for my son, but knowing that there were treatments I could try and actions I could take made it easier. My guilt propelled me to find ways to help him.

We removed dairy from my son's diet the day our therapist told us that it might help. Within two days, his eye contact was drastically improved. I needed no further reason to also remove gluten from his diet. By the end of the summer, I had learned how to read ingredient lists and make gluten- and casein-free meals at home; I also knew I should probably avoid the processed gluten-free items and eat only whole foods. It was an easy sell for me, since I'd always believed that organic is best and had made all of his baby food myself. I decided that if it was good for my son, it was good for all of us, so it became part of our lifestyle very quickly.

It took me several months to decide how I felt about the vaccination issue. While it was too late for Jack, I had a brand new baby boy to make decisions for now, so I got to work. He had already received the ridiculous hepatitis B vaccine at birth, but I couldn't change that now. By his two-month checkup, I had decided it would be best to do a delayed schedule, so I allowed the DTaP and rotavirus vaccinations, and promised to come back in a month for two more. Instead of returning after that month, I kept doing my research. It was one of the most difficult beliefs to overcome during this whole process— I was surrounded by friends, family, the media, and my own beliefs that these horrid diseases would infect my baby if I didn't stick to the recommended schedule. I asked our pediatrician for advice, I read studies that contradicted other studies, and I searched my heart and mind for what truly felt right to me. During that time my baby received another vaccination for DTaP at four months and Hib at six months. By his nine-month appointment, we were knee deep in supplements, biomed, probiotics, and therapy for Jack. I knew now that vaccinations were not right for my family, and I listened to myself.

I asked our pediatrician if I could delay any more until my son was at least in school. I told her that he was low-risk because he stayed home with me and I planned on extended breast-feeding. She tensed up and asked us to leave her practice. We left without argument, but some part of me felt rejected. I felt very alone; I had no friends who had made this choice at that time, and I didn't like the feeling of being outside the norm. Still, I knew she had done us a favor. This was clearly not a person interested in partnering with me in the interest of my children's health.

Around this time, I discovered the Thinking Moms' Revolution. I read the blog religiously every day, taking comfort in knowing there was a group of parents out there doing the same work and making the same choices I was forced to make. Through Facebook groups, I started to find more like-minded moms who I could talk to about treatments, diets, and therapies, and life started to feel more "normal" again.

Just after Jack's second birthday, we started seeing a DAN! doctor in our town. I felt lucky to have someone so close who could help him recover. As many other moms do, I was exhausting myself with research. I joined email groups, Facebook pages, read blogs, books, and other children's lab tests—trying to become a doctor and a chemist overnight to help my son. I understood most of it— how this vitamin helps that function, how to combine supplements appropriately, what his genetic mutations meant, how to kill yeast, bacteria, and parasites. The problem was I didn't believe that any of these issues were the root cause of his problems. Every time the DAN! doctor sent us home with a new supplement to add in, I felt a huge weight bearing down on me. I knew that if his little body didn't have enough of a particular nutrient, there was a deeper problem, one that would not be solved by giving him a synthetic version of it. We did a round of antifungals, along with a ton of probiotics and supplements, including B12 injections, and saw almost no improvement. We considered chelation and parasite protocols. My gut told me this was not the way for us, and this time I listened.

I started to understand that the stress we had caused him through his birth and experiences as a baby needed to be removed at a deeper level. For us it wasn't about metals, or parasites, or yeast. These issues were just symptoms of greater disease and dysfunction in the body.

Our kids have problems with all of those things, but I firmly believe that our bodies should be able to balance themselves when they're given the right environment.

Homeopathy entered my world in March 2013, when my son was two and a half. Every time I saw it mentioned in one of my autism groups, I felt compelled to look into it. I did not fully understand how it worked, but I went with my instinct and made appointments with two different providers, which I cancelled when it just didn't feel right. Finally, I found Rudi Verspoor. At that point I couldn't find anyone who had worked with him, but when I read about his practice something really resonated with me.

The first time I talked to Rudi was over a year ago. I listened to him explain that stress and trauma create disease and imbalances in our bodies, but that Heilkunst (the medical system that he practices) can systematically remove these traumas. He told me that most cases take about two years to resolve, depending on the complexity of the situation. We were to create a timeline of my son's traumatic events, starting with the most recent, all the way back to pregnancy. Once those traumas were cleared, Rudi would then treat for the inherited disease patterns, or miasms, that are passed down from our ancestors and affect us all. He warned that there might be negative reactions to some of the remedies my son would take, but that it was all part of the healing process, likening it to the process of tearing down an old house and building a new one. Finally, an explanation that made sense to me! I knew now that we were on the right path.

We started seeing results within the first six weeks. My son had suffered from low energy and fatigue most of his life, but with Heilkunst he gradually perked up. He was better able to handle his therapy sessions, and he learned to jump and climb quickly. He started gaining new words and putting more words together. He was more engaged with us and more present in our world. Where he had previously wandered away or flat-out resisted social situations with noise, commotion, and strangers, he was now diving right in, watching the other kids and enjoying himself. I knew we had a long road ahead, but seeing all of these positive outcomes showed me that my instinct had been right.

Soon after, I dropped almost all the supplements that he had been on, and his energy improved even more. He still takes a probiotic, digestive enzymes, and cod liver oil, all of which help his digestion and immune system function. I hope someday he won't need these, but for now, it's working well. We've been able to add in some foods again that he had a high IgG reaction to just a year ago, and there's been no apparent downside.

My whole family is being treated with Heilkunst now. We just endured a winter that, based on the constant complaints I heard from friends about their sick children, seemed rough in terms of illness, but my kids never had more than a sniffle. Removing blockages that damage our immune systems and eating whole, organic foods has kept us strong and healthy. I have two younger boys who are completely typical and healthy, and I give much credit to Heilkunst for this.

One of our ongoing challenges has been finding a therapy model that works for Jack. Though I wholeheartedly believe that Heilkunst is ultimately what will bring him back to health, I also feel it is important to actively work on language, motor skills, and social connections. I'm also incredibly impatient for full recovery.

Jack always resisted traditional speech and occupational therapy. We learned some great activities, but it was not time well spent for either of us, as he cried and fought all the things that were challenging for him. After spending a lot of time researching other possible programs that could help, I discovered Becky Blake, founder of Creating Super Kids. She travels around the world to families' homes to set up individualized programs for their children. Having raised a child with autism herself, she spent the last twenty years learning techniques to help their brains and bodies work together better. Becky has developed a model for removing stress, strengthening motor skills, improving language and communication, correcting digestive issues, and more. It's truly amazing that she has figured out how to put together so many different therapies and methods to help children of all abilities. Even better, her theory that stress is the main cause of autism and related disorders corresponds perfectly with Heilkunst and seems to work in much the same way, albeit on a different level.

Within a few days of starting Becky's program, my son was already speaking more. He was more observant, telling me what he sees and what he wants more frequently. His body seemed less out of balance, and he loved the activities that she set up for us, which included music, massage, and games that help improve his attention. He became better able to imitate body movements and control himself.

About a year ago we were introduced to the IonCleanse by A Major Difference. Within the first sixty days of use, Jack's ATEC score dropped nineteen points and I saw serious language gains. Nothing we had done before this showed such a massive change in a short time period. We continue to use the IonCleanse, though not as religiously as before, but I believe it is helping my son to continue his detoxification.

Jack is currently in a semi-structured special education program at our local school. He spends part of his day in the general education room and has lots of friends there. We have been fortunate to find teachers and therapists there who believe that he can recover and are willing to give him the resources he needs to do so. He just finished kindergarten and will move on to first grade in the fall; he can read, do math, and is starting to write. I am so proud of the progress he made this past year!

I have incredible hope for Jack and for our future as a family right now. He has taught me so much about life in the short time he's been on this earth. Our family is stronger and healthier because of him. Most days I feel as though my son is healing me rather than the other way around. I wish that his life was easier and that he hadn't had to endure so much trauma, illness, and frustration, and I would give anything to take all that away from him. But I can't say that I regret anything. I made the best choices for him that I knew to make at the time. When we know better, we do better—and I wouldn't know better if it weren't for my sweet little guy. So do your best, learn everything you can, and above all, *trust yourself.* Your instinct will never lead you astray, but sometimes it can be hard to hear over all of the noise we have to sort through. Learn to hear that voice inside your head, and do what it says to do. You are wiser than you know.

5

Spartan
Treating Today's Medical Autism Is Possible

M Y INTENT IS TO SPEAK STRAIGHT TO YOUR HEARTS, ESPECIALLY to the hearts of mothers with newly diagnosed children. I want you to know that I know how you're feeling right now—lost, alone, and sad. I've been there. I can remember exactly what it felt like in July 2011, sitting across from the naval hospital physician being told these words: "Autism. New normal. Get him ABA therapy, occupational therapy, speech therapy." Not once was anything mentioned about the underlying medical symptoms of today's autism. When I questioned the doctor about my son's horrific constipation, I was told it was just "part of the autism," that diet modification often doesn't work, and that other alternative treatments could be dangerous. At the time, we were stationed in Okinawa, Japan, because my husband was a Marine. The first step in our journey was to return to the United States through a process called a tour conversion.

It took about six months for the tour conversion to go through, and it felt like an eternity. Once we were settled in our new home,

I started my action plan. I refused to let this illness have my son. He was not neurodiverse; he was very sick. I was very fortunate to have spoken to a fellow military spouse who put me in contact with one of the best DAN! doctors in Southern California. By this time, my son was two and a half years old, and I was more than eager to get the ball rolling. One of the first books I read while waiting for our appointment with our new physician was Dr. Kenneth Bock's *Healing the New Childhood Epidemics*. I had heard of Dr. Bock when I worked at a radiology facility in Kingston, New York. How ironic that I would end up needing his information ten years later. As I read each page of his book, I became more and more certain that my son's autism was treatable.

It was almost one year after Connor's diagnosis that we had the first meeting with my son's new physician in June 2012. It ended up being more than I could have hoped for. I was treated with utmost respect, and my belief that indeed my son's underlying issues could be treated was validated. We ran extensive blood, stool, and urine analyses on him, and what they showed was both informative and heartbreaking. My son had horrific gut damage, a depleted immune system, mitochondrial issues, vitamin D deficiency, and a high viral load.

After absorbing all of the results, I had renewed determination to get my child back. Almost one year later, we finally had a game plan in place. The first thing we addressed was healing Connor's damaged gut. With simple diet modifications, his digestion got better, and one of his symptoms—his hand flapping—decreased. After that, we started treating each ailment one by one, and he continued to come back to us. It wasn't until almost one year of healing these issues that we then started to implement other therapies.

One of the biggest reasons I decided to actively write about my son is that I want you to know that you have choices, many choices, regarding treatment for your child. You don't have to accept it when a doctor sits in front of you and tells you that your child was born this way when you know better. Seek out alternative treatments such as biomedical therapies, homeopathy, and chiropractic care. It may all seem daunting at first, or maybe too costly, but what is more important than your child's health? Instead of reading poems about Holland, I want you to research Bernard Rimland and exhaust every single resource available.

This year, the CDC just released their new autism numbers. One in sixty-eight. They made the announcement on the very same day my son was officially released from his IEP for special education. He has recovered. As I sat in front of the therapists and they signed off on my son's capability to stay on par with his peers, my first feeling was to rejoice, but the joy was quickly replaced by the sadness of those new numbers.

This has got to stop! It's up to us as mothers to protect our children. We are their biggest advocates. You can beat this; you can pull your child out of the throes of today's medical autism. We are here for you every single step of the way and on the other side in a place called recovery.

6

Rocky
Eye of the Tiger

"Noah."

"NOO-AH."

"NOAH!!!"

I clap my hands in front of his face. My heart seems to stop beating. The room closes in on me as panic sets in. I've lost him again. My body tenses, and I continue to watch and wait. Holding the phone in a viselike grip, my knuckles turn white. I suddenly remember my friend Diane is still on the other end.

"What happened?" she asks.

"I don't know, he just stares off and doesn't respond. It's like he's unconscious, but his eyes are still open," I explain.

"How often does this happen?"

"All the time, all day long."

Noah is back with me again, sitting in his highchair, staring at Elmo on the TV singing the hotdog song as he picks up a piece of waffle with his fingers and puts it in his mouth. I slowly exhale. I am able to breathe again.

The next morning is our eighteen-month wellness appointment. When he was fifteen months old, our local regional center diagnosed Noah with a global developmental delay and a wide gait. And when Noah was seventeen months, our occupational therapist added sensory processing disorder and hypotonia (low muscle tone). As a part of this diagnostic process, we would have to also rule out apraxia, a disorder of motor planning that affects speech and movement. Dr. P. (our pediatrician) pops into the room a few minutes later: "Hey guys! I will need you to fill out the M-CHAT (Modified Checklist for Autism in Toddlers) today." Soon, all trace of Dr. P.'s usual humor and pleasant demeanor begins to fade, replaced by a look of concern as he measures Noah's head. His head size has grown from the 25th percentile at twelve months to the 90th percentile at eighteen months. My husband Jason and I exchange nervous glances.

I complete the M-CHAT and hand it to Dr. P. He scores it and frowns. He is from Israel, and until now I had always found his accent charming. But now, it is foreboding. "Hmm. Noah has failed the M-CHAT. I am going to refer you to a neurologist to test for autism." Everyone becomes silent. Growing up in a large Italian family, I am accustomed to everyone talking loudly in an effort to be heard. I am not comfortable with silence. I hate the silence.

Later that day, I walk into Noah's nursery to wake him up from his nap and find him carefully walking a circular path in his crib, rhythmically humming. He no longer looks up at me as I approach him. Is this new? Or am I viewing my child differently now because I think he may have autism? He seems unaware of my presence. A feeling of emptiness envelops my heart. "Noah . . . Noah . . . NOOAAH," I call to him. No response. "Why won't you look at me?" He focuses on his path. He methodically places one foot in front of the other, like a tightrope walker tuning out the world, intent on not falling into the abyss.

My despair increases as I fear I have lost a little more of him this day. His two words—"mama" and "da-da"—are replaced by a strange, self-soothing sound. There is no babbling or baby talk. He is smacking the back of his head and jerking his head up and to the side. Is this autism? Does he even know I am here with him right now?

The next morning, I spend several hours with our ABA therapist in our living room, asking Noah to sit down in his chair, hoping he will make eye contact. The transitions into the gated play area for his sessions are unbearable for both of us. His therapist sits in front of him, blocking any chance of escape. I watch my son bravely struggle to overcome his fears caused by an oversensitive nervous system. Noah collapses to the floor. He wails, kicks, then grabs my legs, unable to enter the play area. These meltdowns are excruciating and occur at every transition. I stand behind Noah and pick him up. He grabs a handful of my hair and yanks in desperation. His body goes rigid as I place him into the session and frantically peel his hands off of me. "Just pick him up and place him into the play area, and leave him . . . ignore the behavior," I am told. As soon as he calms down, I am told to come back in. "Tell him to sit down." I am paralyzed by fear. I cannot do it. I am afraid to tell my son to sit down because I know it will trigger another meltdown. And again from the therapist, "You need to remove the emotion. Ignore his behaviors." Just like my son is relearning basic skills that he has lost, I am relearning how to parent my child.

With each session, my heart breaks a little more. I witness Noah's fears growing and his tolerance for the world around him diminishing. It becomes more debilitating for him each day. Noah prefers to stare at the spinning wheels on his toy car rather than actually playing with his toys. He likes to walk his path. To repeatedly throw his toys out of the play area. We are instructed to use behavior momentum, which involves reinforcing positive behaviors and holding back all reinforcement for unwanted behaviors. It does not work. It is unmitigated torture, both to observe in therapy and to attempt on our own. His meltdowns continue to escalate. We are doing the prescribed twenty hours of therapy each week—so why are Noah's behaviors getting worse?

"Autism" is clouding everyone's judgment. No one is considering Noah's health as a contributing factor. Our pediatrician explained to us that "treatment should be based on evidentiary studies," meaning the research would need to show evidence that there is a medical cause for autism. There is no evidence. I countered him: "Yes, but we know this is happening to my son right now . . . and we do not have time to wait. I need to help my son now."

There is chronic diarrhea and nutritional malabsorption caused by candida and clostridia overgrowth in his gut. Eczema. Drool. Food allergies. Seizures. Poor methylation. Mitochondrial dysfunction. Cerebral folate deficiency. Kryptopyrrole, a B6 and zinc deficiency that causes symptoms similar to schizophrenia. High oxalates causing lethargy bordering on hypothyroidism. Low sulfate. High nagalase. Reflux. Noah will eventually be diagnosed with all these conditions. The medical studies are beginning to confirm these health issues in subsets of kids with autism.

Unfortunately, our pediatrician was not current on the latest research. Noah was suffering from severe abdominal pain. His nervous system was badly damaged. If the medical community is not looking deeper at the cause of his behaviors, how are the ABA providers supposed to know to take physical pain into consideration? No one is looking or thinking beyond the behaviors. No one seems to be thinking at all. Is it productive to force Noah to work through his pain? Are we doing more damage in the process? I know something is very wrong with my son beyond the "autism."

Following our ABA session, I feed Noah lunch and then drive him thirty minutes to an OT (occupational therapy) appointment with Tim. (Noah began receiving OT following his diagnosis of sensory processing disorder. He was later diagnosed with dyspraxia, a

neurological condition and disorder of the nervous system charac-
terized by difficulty in motor planning that affected his speech and
fine and gross motor skills.) I sigh as I look at the pond between the
parking lot and Tim's office. The path is a good distance with many
small stone steps to navigate. I have to carefully maneuver those steps
while carrying a resisting and agitated eighteen-month-old Noah who
is unable to sit upright in his stroller. We do not yet know that Noah
has mitochondrial dysfunction that on a bad day will cause him to
have low energy and stamina. Noah can no longer walk from the
car to Tim's office. He is unbearably heavy and slips out of my arms,
which are beginning to grow numb. He hates to be touched or picked
up, making the trek from the car to the office much more difficult.

And, as if to push the limits of my sanity, Noah picks this
moment to unload number two. At first, I think I am okay because,
yup, I am a prepared mommy and I double diapered him today.
Unfortunately for both of us, two diapers are no match for this load.
It is massive and explosive and leaks through both diapers, onto his
clothing and onto me. By the time I arrive at Tim's office, there is
diarrhea all over me and Noah. I feel like I am going to lose it. *Shit!*
Shit! SHIT! I hate my life. And then: *Oh, God. And I am sick again?*
My cold has turned into bronchitis. I have the chills, I am coughing
from deep down in my chest, and I am so very, very tired.

I make it to Tim's office and run past the receptionist, already
ten minutes late. I head straight to the back room to the changing
table. I brace myself as I do my best to gently lay Noah down. He
refuses. *No. No! NO!!! You've got to be kidding me. Please, please, let*
me change your diaper. Noah fights me like his life depends on it. He
cries, screams, pulls my hair, punches and kicks me—anything to
avoid being laid down in that position. What the hell? How is he so
strong? Shit is everywhere—literally. Why are you doing this to me?
YOU ARE GOING TO MISS YOUR THERAPY. Please, PLEASE,
stop fighting me! PLEASE!!! Oh, God, I can't think straight, my head
feels foggy. *Why won't you let me change your diaper?*

Noah suffered from severe vestibular dysfunction—the feeling of being at the top of a roller coaster the moment you are about to plunge downward. Noah was experiencing this all the time, which also made sitting upright in his car seat and his stroller terrifying for him.

Completely spent, shit smeared on my clothing and in my hair, I carry Noah into Tim's office. Tim looks at me with a deep level of compassion as I hand Noah over to him as if he is the anchor in our makeshift relay team. He takes over for me for at least an hour. Noah cries the entire time. He is unable to sit in the swing, touch the shaving cream, or find the floor in front of his feet as Tim walks with him, giving him joint compression.

In addition to vestibular dysfunction, Noah also has tactile dysfunction (oversensitivity to touch) and proprioceptive dysfunction (lack of body awareness). For Noah, sensory integration dysfunction triggers excessive emotional reactions. Leaning against the wall in the large therapy room, I let myself slide slowly to the floor. I am emotionally depleted, torn between the urge to end Noah's session, unable to bear his cries, and the urge to postpone the inevitable battle of getting Noah organized and back across the pond and into his car seat. At this point, it's more than I can bear. I just want to lie down, close my eyes, and have someone else take over. For today at least.

Jason and I are silent the next afternoon as we sit in the waiting room for our appointment with Dr. N., the neurologist. Fortunately, there is a train table to keep Noah entertained while we wait. Noah is obsessed with trains. We are alone with our thoughts. We are eventually led back to Dr. N.'s office, where he asks us various questions and tests Noah. Nothing can prepare you for what comes next, even if you already suspect it.

"Your son has autism." Just like that.

"I don't believe it. Why is it autism? Why not sensory processing disorder?"

Dr. N. smiles and replies, "Guys, this is a good thing. It's autism. Now you know."

No bedside manner. I hate him. I need someone at whom I can direct my rage, and it may as well be him. Looking back, I am grateful that this neurologist was direct with us. And he was right; someone had to be. But, at that moment, this future warrior mom continued to argue with him as he insisted Noah's autism must be genetic: "But, no one in our family has anything like this." Dr. N. tears out a sheet of paper from his notebook and writes out a "prescription" for twenty-five hours of therapy per week that includes ABA, speech, OT, and PT. "Oh, and some of my clients have had success with the GFCF diet, but there is no evidence to back it up. And document the staring spells. They could be seizures, but I don't like to do EEGs unnecessarily. And schedule a follow-up appointment in six months." It would take us three years, two DAN! doctors, a nutritionist, and a second neurologist to get what were, in fact, seizures under control.

I am devastated and cannot stop crying. For my son and for my family. When Noah was born, I had the usual hopes and dreams for him. But autism had suddenly taken these hopes and dreams hostage. Now I wonder if he will ever talk, go to a regular school, be able to make friends. I resolve to give my son his childhood and, ultimately, his life back. I keep asking questions, knowing deep inside that there are answers different than what we have been told. There have to be. That night I make a promise to Noah that I will never give up on him. I cannot sleep and am googling for information late into the night.

I sit in on Noah's next session with Tim, taking notes as we discuss everything that has transpired over the past few days. Tim mentions that he is working on a study that looks at the growing number of children with sensory issues in areas of high fungal rates, suggesting that mold may be a consideration. Tim also loans me his copy of *Children with Starving Brains* by Jaquelyn McCandless. After the session, he writes out a list of labs and biomarkers to bring to our doctor.

Jason hires a mold inspector to come to our house the next day. The inspector opens a small panel in the wall of Noah's nursery and discovers a large amount of black mold. Samples reveal a high level of aspergillus. We later learn that our landlord had had shoddy plumbing work done shortly before our tenancy began. Our first DAN! doctor will test for mycotoxins in Noah's urine and find a high amount of ochratoxin, a biotoxin derived from aspergillus and penicillin.

Later that evening, as we sit down to discuss the possibility that mold may be contributing to Noah's developmental delays and health issues, I feel like the room is closing in on me. What the hell? We chose this house! It was our responsibility to ensure a safe environment for Noah. If we had been more careful, our son would be fine. We were responsible and wanted desperately to fix it. Was it possible to do so?

Over the ensuing days, between finding a new place to live and shuttling Noah to and from various therapy appointments, I begin to wonder—could the vaccinations also be contributing to Noah's condition? Through conversations with Tim, I begin to realize that perhaps there is not one single contributing factor, but rather a combination of exposure to biotoxins (mold) and subjecting a weakened immune system to multiple strains of live viruses (vaccinations). Was Noah's body overburdened with environmental toxins?

I call Dr. B., a DAN! doctor, and schedule our first appointment at the California Integrative Hyperbaric Center in Irvine. At that first visit, I meet David Kartzinel (the son of Dr. Jerry Kartzinel, Jenny McCarthy's coauthor for the book *Healing and Preventing Autism*) in the front office, and he gives me the 411 on biomedical treatment and talks to me about vaccines and environmental toxins. I feel at home and am overcome by emotion. David hands me a TACA (parent-support non-profit organization called Talk About Curing Autism) card that says: "My child's behavior may be disturbing to you. My child is not spoiled or misbehaving. My child has autism."

On the back: "Autism is a devastating biological and neurological disorder that can affect individuals in different areas." The card lists the five areas: communication, social, behavior, sensory, and medical. As I read it, tears roll down my face, as I realize that these TACA folks are describing my son. For the first time since starting down this path in search of answers, I feel as though someone got it just right—someone is seeing the whole picture, the whole child. This is when it hits me like a ton of bricks how significantly our medical community—the people I trusted to fix this—have let me down. Autism is not genetic. Noah's autism is caused by toxins in his environment that are poisoning him and destroying his health. I take the card with me as I am called back to Dr. B.'s office. This is the first true step to recovery, and I will never look back.

It is Thanksgiving week 2013. It is the three-year anniversary of our diagnosis. I am driving with the four-and-a-half-year-old Noah in the back seat. It is a beautiful day. My parents are on their way to our house to join us for the holiday. This will be our first "paleo" Thanksgiving so that everyone can enjoy a meal together as a family.

I feel healthy and energized. Since beginning our journey of recovery, I have changed my diet, introduced weekly infrared sauna sessions for detox, and added essential oils and herbs and supplements for extra support. I stop at a light and use the opportunity to look at Noah in the rear-view mirror. He is a truly beautiful child. I am momentarily mesmerized and think at that moment that he is absolutely perfect. I take the moment to ask, "Noah, what are you most thankful for this Thanksgiving?"

He brushes aside a strand of his long blond hair and looks up at me with his steel-blue eyes. "You, Mommy. I am thankful for you." As tears fill my eyes, I turn my attention back to the road. Our journey of healing is not over. But I know that we are heading the right way.

7

Crush

Inspiring Strangers, Incompetent Doctors, Incredible Kids

I REMEMBER THE DAY MY DAUGHTER CALI RECEIVED HER DIAGnosis; the moment is burned into my soul. The words said to us that day will never be far from my thoughts. Seething words that shatter parents' dreams just rolling off the neurologist's tongue as if this were just an everyday conversation about the weather. These phrases would be repeated over and over by medical professional after medical professional so many times in the first few years that the words are never far from my thoughts, even today.

Your daughter has autism. There is no known cure, no known cause; it will not get better, and it is likely to get worse. She will never speak. She will never have friends. She will never be able to function in a normal school setting. There really is nothing to do. She is a danger to herself and others. We can try medication, but there is no guarantee. I don't know how to explain to you that this is just something that goes along with autism. We can't help you. You need to consider putting her in an institution.

You need to consider putting her in an institution!

We were told that by the time Cali turned four, we should just stop bothering. Cali was never going to be anything more than what she was, and it was time to walk away. But this made no sense to me. How do you tell someone that there is no hope, and in the same conversation admit that you don't even know what is wrong? How do you walk away from a child, just give up on her, when you haven't even tried to look for answers? How do you say there is no possibility if you don't try? There are a number of things I took away from those conversations: disgust, anger, sadness, frustration. But never did I leave an appointment and think they were right. Never.

Looking back, I know we didn't start out here. We started out with a baby that by all evaluations was deemed a perfectly healthy child (although now it's clear that this was likely not the case). There were issues before pregnancy (environmental toxins, family health history, medications) that should have been considered. There were issues for myself during pregnancy (illness, adverse reaction to the Rh shot, strange rashes) that were dismissed by my team of providers. There were issues at birth (delayed birth, lack of oxygen, medication, poor medical care) that are inexcusable. And there were issues *after* birth (surgery and health issues for myself, and food intolerances, GI problems, and reflux for my daughter) that were swept under the rug as normal.

And yet somehow, with all of that being said, Cali was a beautiful, happy baby who had normal scores at birth and normal well-baby visits. Everyone said she was doing great. By all appearances, she was our perfect, amazing little angel. We followed every guideline, listened to every word of advice the doctors gave, read every baby book, and took her on time to every doctor's appointment. She smiled, rolled over, responded to her name, walked, played, and started talking, all on time or early. Life was good. And we were proud parents who were completely unaware of the storm that was brewing, the pieces piling up, and the life changes that were shortly to come.

March 1, 2004, was the day that changed everything and would rock life as we knew it. I brought Cali to our trusted pediatrician for her twelve-month well visit. I remember hearing babies crying, and I was trying to keep my daughter distracted by reading books, playing with toys, and smothering her cute little face in kisses so she would giggle. We weighed, measured, talked about how adorable she was, and I signed the papers for her shots. And then I held my child and told her it was going to be okay while they injected her with the MMR and varicella vaccinations. And within hours my beautiful, smiling daughter was gone. Encephalopathy from vaccination. Those are the words that are listed on her records. The promise of it being okay was forever stuck in my heart. It wouldn't be okay that day. Actually, it wouldn't be okay for many years. The storm had hit, the tipping point was toppled, and our world would never be the same.

I retreated to my bathroom floor, shut the door, and tried to breathe. Sitting on the cold tile, tears running down my face, I prayed (often begged) for answers. I could not even grasp the idea of looking ahead or believing in hope. I was stuck in survival mode. Cali was three and half, and the days of before were barely recognizable. Hurting so deeply, I looked into those same beautiful eyes for a glimmer that showed that Cali even knew who I was; I searched for any signs of the child that used to be.

Our days were on repeat. I spent hours pacing the house, picking up objects and trying to find something that would satisfy the screams. I wrapped my arms around her so tightly and rocked her because letting go meant she would harm herself by throwing her body into walls or slamming her head against the floor. Our fourth copy of *Aladdin* played in the background from her favorite scene because it was the only thing she seemed to hear. Alarms were installed on the windows and doors just in case she found a second that we were distracted and decided to elope. We couldn't leave home or be around new faces because those everyday activities produced an epic meltdown that involved kicking, screaming, biting, or hiding in the closest shrubbery. Our home had become both our safe place and our prison.

There were emergency room visits for hernias, ear infections, strep, GI problems, and injuries that she didn't feel. Tylenol and round after round of antibiotics had become the recommended staple from the physicians. I watched for any sign of the skills that had disappeared; the ones she retained had become so structured that we couldn't sway from routines even an inch. Friends had disappeared, doctors were completely clueless, and our family was trying but unsure how to help. Our marriage was falling apart, we worried about the safety of the baby on the way, and the bills stacked up as autism was an insurance "exclusion" at the time. My world was crashing down around me. Sixteen hours a day of screaming, and that little meltdown spot on the bathroom floor was all I knew to do when she finally rested. We felt alone and without hope, praying for miracles. Cali was in her own dire world and we had no clue how to get her out.

Miracles sometimes come in the most unusual ways. Cali was four and a half, and little had changed. I had been working from home as a travel specialist, assisting groups in planning vacations. This memorable morning, I headed to the airport to see a group of high school students and their moms off on a trip. I arrived early, checked the departures, and gathered my paperwork for the group. Shortly the travelers began to arrive, and the excitement filled the air. This was a group of fun young women—I enjoyed working with them. The mom who organized the trip was a special education teacher, and we had shared many conversations.

This morning was no different as I welcomed her, and immediately she asked about Cali. As we were chatting, one of the fathers who had brought his daughter to the airport walked over, apologized, and interrupted our conversation. My first thought was that his daughter had forgotten her ticket or he had a question about luggage. Little did I know that he was about to change my life. He explained that he overheard our conversation, and that he didn't mean to interrupt but had to say something. He went on to tell me that I had to speak with his wife, and that he couldn't give me all the details because it was his wife who had really done it all, but that his daughter was also once diagnosed with autism. He shared that his wife had done all these "alternative things" and then turned to point out his daughter.

She was in my departing group. I had no clue. Here before me stood this beautiful young lady, surrounded by friends and giggling about the plans for their trip. At one time, she was supposedly like my daughter? I knew this young lady from our planning meetings and was aware that she was graduating and heading to college out of state on academic and athletic scholarships. She was popular, smart, had a boyfriend, and spent her free time like any other teenager. And she had a proud and nervous father willing to walk up to me and share with me the first glimmer of hope I had in years. A random kind man, who would change everything in a matter of one small conversation. My miracle.

We didn't have time for more than those few words as the group was due for their flight. I watched the girls and moms head to the gate, and the dad disappeared to his car before I had the chance to get his wife's information. I gathered my stuff and headed to my car. I sat with the engine running, and for the first time in four years, I cried like a baby. Tears of pain, sadness, guilt, anger all pouring down my face as I finally let it all go. Life was about to change again drastically, but this time it would be toward the promise I made to my daughter so many years ago: it would be okay. I drove home and shared this story with my husband, and we set out on the path to change this course that very same day, starting with the basics of dietary changes.

Improvement doesn't happen overnight, but we stayed committed to addressing health issues and treating any underlying medical problems. One day, when Cali was five, I was bringing in the groceries, arms overflowing. I had taken the opportunity to get out alone. I opened the door and Cali looked right at me and said, "Momma!" I dropped every bag I held and stood there for what seemed like hours crying tears of joy, holding her in my arms. Never was a sweeter word said. It wasn't recovery or cure, but it sure as hell was one of the greatest joys of my life.

Life had become easier. Once we changed her diet, things began to shift, and the screams disappeared. The behaviors that once ruled our home were now gone. Cali looked at us again. She found language. She made a friend. She played T-ball. Life wasn't perfect, and we knew we had a ways to go, but our path was paved by those before us, and we knew she was getting better. We became less concerned with what the world had decided for my daughter and focused on what we decided for her. We discovered we were not alone, and we had things to try, and my daughter had a lifetime to prove the doctors wrong.

Fast forward to the first grade. Cali was six years old and about to show the world that she is proof that kids can and do improve when we address autism from a medical framework as opposed to accepting it as some sort of predetermined outcome. I was sitting in a school meeting room, awaiting the arrival of those involved in the IEP process. (The IEP is an individualized education plan given to address the needs of an individual who is not on peer level academically. A team strategically addresses areas that need additional help/resources and formulates a plan to help the student achieve "goals.") Our team consisted of representatives from the school district, therapists, and teachers. The stress of these meetings was long gone, as I had become accustomed to them. The team members evaluate and tell me how far behind my child still is. We set goals, and I try to find the strength to not focus on all the things she could not do, but instead appreciate the things we have accomplished. But this meeting was different. As the binders opened and pens came out, I heard something about removing her IEP.

The shock rippled through me. I realized they were telling me that she was, by all evaluations, on the same level as her peers. I had no idea what to say or do, because I was prepared for the way these meetings usually went. One foot in front of the other, no looking backward, celebrating every small accomplishment . . . that's how we roll. And yet, here I sat, hearing that my once nonverbal child, whose evaluations showed her at a nine- to twelve-month-old's skill levels after the regression and who, according to the doctors, would never make it in school, was being removed from services because she didn't need them. The pieces were coming together.

In 2010, I took my daughter back to her original diagnosing neurologist. I have to admit I may have done it with an agenda. Cali was eight, and we were moving across the country to where my husband was being stationed for military duty. I probably needed to get all of our medical records in order, but mainly I just wanted to show the neurologist how totally fucking wrong he was.

It was clear from the moment he walked into the room that he didn't really remember my daughter. He asked why we were there, and I explained that we wanted to have our last annual exam as we were moving. He asked my daughter to hop up on to the examination table, and she walked over and bounced right up there smiling. As he examined her eyes and tracking, she casually told him how she was a straight-A student, and that she loved sports and playing with her friends. I could see the confusion growing, but he said nothing and continued her exam, measured her head, checked her reflexes, and listened for signs of repetitive language. He asked about her emotions, her health, and life overall. After a thorough exam, he finally helped her down from the table and told her she could play with the toys he had in the room while we talked. I gave Cali a smile and walked over to his desk.

It was the dreaded desk that we had sat behind so many times over the years. The desk where he had told me five years ago that Cali had autism. The same desk where he scratched out a list of things to *not* consider as causes of autism. The same desk where he told me there was no known cause (yeah, right) and no known cures (ha!). The same desk where he sat a year later and he told me she would never get better and would likely get worse. The same desk where he uttered the sentence: "You need to consider putting her in an institution." The same desk where he told me she would never speak, never have friends, never make it in a school setting. The same desk where he said none of those "alternative things" would help and we would just be wasting time that we could use to deal with reality. The desk from hell. But not that day, not ever again.

He opened her file and began scanning through the notes. He read them out loud, phrases and words like "danger to herself and others," "violent," "psychotic," "severe," "institution," and "medications." I wanted to laugh out loud at the things he wrote knowing he had to be wondering if he had the right records. I just smiled and listened. And then he closed the file and said, "Well, she sure seems to be doing well on the medication." I said very nicely, "Oh, she isn't on any medication." He opened the folder to look again and said, "I prescribed medication back in 2007 to address some of these issues." I explained to him that while he had indeed suggested that, my husband and I opted to go a different route. Confused but still unwilling to admit that we had found answers that he didn't provide, he started to applaud the ABA therapy. Again, I explained that while he had suggested that, we opted to treat the medical issues instead. No ABA either. Frustrated with the conversation, he picked up his pen and asked what we had done. And then he started writing.

I explained to him that we investigated those so-called alternatives, such as diet and treating underlying issues. I added with a big, fat smile, "You know, all that stuff you advised us against—biomedical care." And I continued, "Within a matter of months, we had eye contact, no more meltdowns, no behavior problems, and she was in school. Within a year, she was caught up to her peers, and within two she was testing in the top 1 percent of the country. She has friends, plays sports, is not in pain, and is happy."

He looked back into the folder, took a deep breath, closed the folder again, and then leaned across the desk from hell and said, "I need to shake your hand." I didn't know whether to fall out of the chair, cry, or punch him in the face. He continued, "If I could bottle up what you have done, I would be rich." And because I came there determined to show him this child, whom he long ago dismissed—and the truth about hope—I said, "You can. You can tell every parent who comes here from now on that there is hope, there are answers. Do not let them walk out of this office believing the things you told us over the past six years." And we left the office and headed home floating on the belief that maybe, just maybe, this neurologist would be the start of other families seeking answers, believing in the possibilities, and knowing there was so much more.

Even looking back seven years later is very difficult. It seems like I am looking back on someone else's life. Today there are very few traces of autism. Cali still struggles occasionally with very chaotic or loud places, has some health issues and nutritional deficiencies that we manage, and still can't grasp why people are mean or why doctors aren't helping all the kids who are like she once was. She is a straight-A student, plays sports, and loves theater and film. She has best friends and sleepovers, and she covers her walls in posters of the latest boy bands. She teaches her peers about what autism is like and loves to explain why nobody should move to Mississippi because of their limited vaccine rights. She has the biggest heart and shows more empathy and compassion than most adults. She writes stories and loves helping other kids with special needs. She is her sister's best friend, and their giggles are priceless. She never misses a moment to say how amazing parents fighting for their kids are, or how thankful she is that we never gave up.

She will change this world, I have no doubt. She changes lives every day. She inspires people, and she brings hope. While I know every story won't look like ours, I know that every little change, every step forward is so worth it. Hope is there every single day. I struggled with that for some time, but it was there, it just needed a push. I needed someone or something to remind me that we were stronger than we knew, that we were filled with courage and fight, and that nothing could stop us. I needed to be reminded that life was what we made of it. That it is okay to look forward, even if it's just a little glance, to remind us to keep going.

I have to thank others before us, those who were in the trenches, who pushed the science, demanded the answers, fought for change, and inspired us. The strangers in the airport, the friends online, the doctors who get it, the parents going through the same struggle that many of us don't even know, and the loved ones who stand beside us. I could never have done this without all of you. You did this. You helped me keep that promise I made so many years ago on that awful day. It will be okay.

Not only does life look different today for our family and for my daughter, but my own personal journey is nothing I imagined. Today my focus is on others, on being someone else's stranger. It's come full circle for me. I fight now for those who are sitting on their cold bathroom floor trying to find a way to survive the day, who can't imagine their life ever being different, who haven't yet found the strength inside themselves, and for those who can't bear to hear any more comments about no answers or no hope. To those parents who today will be told it won't get better, I say, *it will!* We are friends, given to each other, determined to change this world, and we have each other's back. Nothing will stop us now. We are healing, and we are finding hope. We are changing the course of medicine and science.

We are in a revolution! And we are going to CRUSH those who stand in the way of our children!

8

Beaker
What I Now Know

THE GASTROENTEROLOGIST KNELT DOWN ON THE FLOOR, LOOKED MY then one-year-old, nonverbal, failure-to-thrive daughter in the eye, and said, "Sweetie, there is nothing wrong with you. You need to just tell your mommy to quit worrying about you so much, you are just fine." Then he turned to leave the room, looked back, and said, "Get her off your breast milk, mom, and get her drinking cow's milk so she finally gains some weight." And the door shut behind him.

In that moment, I not only accepted that I was alone, but that I alone was going to have to get to the bottom of what was happening to my baby girl. My daughter had just turned a year old, and none of the five pediatric specialists (two gastrointestinal doctors, two allergists, and a pediatrician) whom we consulted could find anything "wrong." However, they also offered *no* explanation, and, more importantly, *no* relief for her pain or other symptoms that worsened with each passing day.

For those first two glorious weeks of her life, my sweet baby girl nursed beautifully. She slept, she cuddled, she napped—she was the picture of health and perfection. I even recall my husband joking on the phone with his brother (who had two sons already), encouraging him to "try for a third one." He said, "It is so worth it, dude, this girl thing is so peaceful!" Our first child, five at the time, was a boy full of noise, spunk, and energy.

By her third week of life, everything had changed. Our daughter began to scream. Not cry, not whimper, but scream. By her six-week well-baby visit, the screaming had gotten worse and her periods of sleep had become shorter and shorter with each passing day. Her obvious discomfort required that we hold her upright for any of us to get any rest at all. She breastfed nonstop and was voracious (almost like she could not get enough, ever). The pediatrician said it must be colic and sent us home saying it would soon pass. Before leaving, though, she had her nurse inject my daughter with four vaccines containing numerous antigens and an oral live virus, for good measure.

What I Now Know (WINK)

1. There is no such thing as colic. Colic is a made-up term left over from the 1950s that has little medical significance other than to describe a fussy baby. Sound familiar? Kind of like autism is a made-up term to describe a child who doesn't look you in the eyes and has repetitive behaviors. Some of the causes of "colic" include reflux, food intolerance (often the major culprit is milk), "rare" metabolic disorders, and weak muscles that control the LES (lower esophageal sphincter). (See the book *Colic Solved.*)

The "colic" was unrelenting, and we were soon back to see the pediatrician, who began us on what I call reflux-med roulette: Zantac, Prevacid, Bethanechol, back to Prevacid, add a little Carafate, put in some more Zantac. We would see a glimmer of relief with each new med change, and we would hold our breath only to see it evaporate a few days later. More shots at four months, right on schedule, and then six-month shots—all six of them. Then came the vinegar-smelling poopy diapers. The blood-curdling screams continued, and no one in our house was sleeping at all.

Our pediatrician finally agreed at seven months that we might need to see a GI doctor. So off we went to the first GI consult. Puzzled but intrigued, the doctor set out to help us figure things out. He changed some meds with no improvement, changed some foods we were feeding her with no improvement, and then started me on a breast-feeding elimination diet. First out went milk (which was not too bad—since I despise the stuff, it was already mostly out of my diet). Then he pulled eggs from my diet, then soy—and for the first time in months our baby girl was calm and peaceful.

Being the engineer and scientist that my husband and I are, we launched into "experimental protocol mode." I grabbed a journal, which became my "lab notebook," and my husband eloquently pronounced, holding a peaceful baby girl for the first time since those first weeks, "Beaker, whatever you did yesterday, whatever you ate, you have to repeat it for fourteen days. If it is the food, then we will know for sure."

Easier said than done. So for fourteen days I ate the same thing every day: oatmeal, brown rice, ground turkey, mixed vegetables, and a few fruits. I was distraught (not to mention *so* hungry). I went to a La Leche meeting in desperate need of validation and support from anyone who knew anything about breast-feeding an allergic child. Instead, what I found was a leader who told me it was impossible for a child to be allergic or even sensitive to a mother's milk and I just needed to eat anything I wanted and feed her whatever I was eating. These words crushed me. Once again, I was looking for support, but found quite the contrary. I was discouraged at that moment, but looking back, it led me to another WINK moment.

2. It is very possible for a baby to be "allergic" to breast milk if the baby's mother is eating foods that the baby cannot digest well

or to which they are intolerant. Later, I would find out a version of the breast-feeding elimination diet we had created by trial and error is called a TED diet (Total Elimination Diet, discussed on the Dr. Sears website). I also found a very supportive group of moms who knew the ins and outs of breast-feeding an allergic/food sensitive child on the forum kidswithfoodallergies.org.

The fourteen-day experiment gave us our answer. What we didn't know then was that food was only part of the puzzle. By her first birthday, our daughter was falling off the growth charts (and her very hungry momma was not far behind her). We had a much more peaceful baby, but on the limited diet for both of us, we struggled to find enough "safe" foods to satisfy her body's demands. She also still seemed to have a constant round-the-clock need for food. We consulted a second GI, who sent us into panic mode with his urgent need to "scope her" immediately, declaring that we were witnessing a child with failure to thrive.

An endoscopy and colonoscopy followed. This included heavy sedation for the procedure and biopsy results that the GI doc pronounced normal. This led to his pronouncement that all our daughter needed was cow's milk—the condescending exchange that began this chapter. Then a couple more vaccines for good measure (including her MMR), and our little girl regressed before our eyes. Within two months after the last round of shots, and two weeks after following the GI doctor's orders to wean her to cow's milk, she began banging her head on anything hard she could find . . . including our tile floor. I watched in horror and held her in bear hugs, crying and pleading for her to stop and praying that I could keep her from hurting herself. We stopped the cow's milk immediately, although the doctor claimed there was no way that the milk could be related to the behavior. He stated that this could just be normal toddler behavior, yet if it continued, perhaps she should be evaluated for autism. I immersed myself in research into the late hours of the night, and eventually endless Google scholar,

Pub-Med, and scientific journal searches led me to another WINK moment.

3. Eosinophils in the gut, head banging, and failure to thrive are NOT normal; in fact, they are quite abnormal and cause for great concern in ANY child. What the GI doc failed to acknowledge was that eosinophils (a type of white blood cell that can become active when you have certain allergic diseases, infections, and other medical conditions, according to *MedlinePlus*) are not supposed to be found in anyone's gut, and when they are present in great numbers, they lead to an allergic, inflammatory condition called eosinophilic gastritis. The pathology report showed eosinophils in my daughter's GI tract, but the doc claimed everything was normal . . . oh, and that I was worrying too much. But I wouldn't know just how big an issue this was for another eight months, when a third gastroenterologist we consulted had the biopsy slides re-read and his pathologist found the same thing—eosinophils. The difference was that this GI doctor knew eosinophils were not supposed to be in a child's gut, or anywhere in their GI tract for that matter!

Head banging is not normal and can be one sign of autism or other developmental disorders in the form of self-injurious behavior. Possible causes include seizures, neurotransmitter imbalances, food intolerances, or genetic conditions. (Source: Autism Research Institute.)

And finally, failure to thrive: "Failure to thrive (FTT) is a term used to describe inadequate growth or the inability to maintain growth, usually in early childhood. It is a sign of under nutrition, and because many biologic, psychosocial, and environmental processes can lead to under nutrition, FTT should never be a diagnosis unto itself" (Source: American Academy of Family Physicians). Well, that certainly does not sound normal or healthy for any kid. "A diagnosis unto itself" is exactly what we got until the next leg of the journey began.

At this point, we were close to giving up on the medical profession. None of what they were telling us seemed to make any sense, and the advice we were given certainly wasn't improving the situation. In many incidences, the treatments they were recommending were actually making our daughter's condition worse. So, we sought the advice of a naturopath who had experience with autistic children. We hoped to find guidance on what we could feed our daughter since she was reacting to so many foods, both gastrointestinally and neurologically.

This doctor ordered a stool test and gave us some dietary advice. He confirmed our suspicion and concerns about vaccination and got her started on a probiotic. The stool test came back positive for Clostridium difficile toxin A and B (C. diff). How the heck did my fifteen-month-old get a bacterial GI infection that is common in hospitals, the elderly, or those who have been on frequent antibiotics when she had not had an antibiotic or hospitalization at this point in her not-so-elderly life? In trying to figure out what this meant for my daughter, I consulted with her pediatrician and GI doc for clarification, and this is the conflicting information I received.

Her pediatrician told me babies are carriers of C. diff and never tested for it until after two years of age, so not to be worried about the result that the naturopath had told us was concerning and needed treatment. The following day, after seeing her pediatrician, we see the gastroenterologist, who walks in the room and declares, "She has C. diff."

"She does?" I question, explaining what the pediatrician had just told me. He proceeds to tell me the test was for the toxin, meaning that this was the active state of the C. diff, and since she was having chronic diarrhea, this could be the cause. We treated with an herbal treatment the naturopath had recommended, and the C. diff retest results came back normal. I feel a WINK coming on . . .

4. Clostridium difficile (C. diff) overgrowth and toxin is bad—very bad—and, according to the FDA, has been recently linked

to use of reflux medications (proton pump inhibitors such as the Prevacid our daughter had been taking). Remember that reflux roulette that the docs were playing? Ummm, yeah. Awesome. Oh, and in mouse models, Clostridia bacterial strains can produce excess propionic acid which, when injected directly into mice, can cause them to look "autistic." (See the study by R.E. Frye et al in *Translational Psychiatry* 3 (2013)). Coincidence? I think not.

I wish the story ended there, but the journey continued. Upon returning from a family vacation when my daughter was almost eighteen months old, we reached what I recall as the bottom. As in rock bottom. Things got worse. Just as we felt we were solving the "mystery," we would find another clue. This particular "clue" came in this form: I was removing some of my nail polish using a non-acetone, alcohol-based remover. My daughter was quietly playing in my closet with my shoes. I had finished a few nails when I heard a blood-curdling scream coming from the adjacent closet. My daughter was lying on her back in a back-bend position, screaming. As I picked her up, she was as stiff as a board. I had no idea what had happened, she had no blood or cuts, and her brother was not in the room, so I could not figure out why she was so upset.

After nearly twenty minutes of trying to calm her down, and two frantic calls to the pediatrician and my husband, she took a sip of water. I had to go to the bathroom, so I took her back into my bathroom with me to keep an eye on her. The minute we stepped back into the doorway of the bathroom, she began to scream and stiffen again. I ran out of the room with her in my arms, and out the front door of our house to fresh air. Within minutes she calmed down. It hit me . . . it was the nail polish remover chemicals, still lingering in the air of the bathroom. Over the next week, our observation and hypothesis would be tested. Similar "behaviors" and screaming ensued when her brother squirted hand sanitizer near her, when we sprayed our countertops with Windex and it evaporated near her, and when we wiped her face with alcohol-containing baby wipes.

When my breath (after an adult beverage) was near her face, she started slapping my mouth. The common ingredient was ethanol. My baby had a severe intolerance to inhaled ethanol fumes. How did that happen?

5. The reflux medication Zantac (Ranitidine) in the syrup/ liquid form (for children and babies) contains *alcohol* (ethanol). "Zantac Syrup contains 7.5% w/v alcohol. Each spoonful (5 mL) of syrup therefore contains almost 400 mg of alcohol. This is equal to the amount of alcohol in one spoonful (5 mL) of wine or two spoonfuls (10 mL) of beer" (Source: Glaxo consumer sheet). So let me get this straight. The American Academy of Pediatrics encourages moms who are breast-feeding to limit alcohol consumption and delay nursing for two hours after consuming alcohol, but the AAP's own member (our pediatrician) handed me a prescription for an equivalent of two spoonfuls of beer (plus some H2 blocker for good measure) a few times a day for my baby? I wish I had been a little less sleep deprived and a little more educated back then to question this, but sadly I was not. We were in survival mode.

The next morning after the reaction to the nail polish remover was my daughter's eighteen-month "well visit." I stayed up the entire night researching ethanol sensitivity and around 2 a.m. came to this conclusion that I wrote to my husband in an email: "We have to push for metabolic testing. Period. Love you . . . goodnight." The next day, I pleaded with our pediatrician to send us to a metabolic specialist. She told me the wait for a geneticist would be over a year, referred us to a neurologist, and offered my daughter another vaccination booster! No thanks, not until you tell me what the hell is happening to my little girl that she cannot tolerate the smell of the rubbing alcohol that you are going to wipe her skin with before you inject her!

The neurologist did the first tests for mitochondrial (mito) disease (blood testing for lactic acid and pyruvic acid), as well as many other conditions. The mito testing came back abnormal, so he repeated the tests two more times. All abnormal. The preliminary biomarkers were positive for mitochondrial disease. While we waited three months to see the mitochondrial specialist, our food discoveries continued.

Our daughter's diet at this point was free of dairy, casein, gluten, and soy. In place of wheat flour, we were baking a ton with almond flour and letting her drink almond milk. On that family vacation I mentioned, we could not find almond milk, so we switched to rice milk for the trip. Upon returning, we went back to almond. She had few, if any, behavioral reaction to foods while on vacation, but upon returning home she began regressing and was miserable. While I was trying to figure out what could be causing her to decline, it dawned on me that maybe the almonds were a clue—there was a connection between all the foods she did not tolerate (the list was mostly made up of highly colored red, orange, and purple fruits and veggies).

Being the geeky chemist that I am, I hypothesized that the food itself might not be the issue; perhaps it was the chemical that they all contained that made them highly colored. After many a Google search, I found it: they were all high in salicylates or sali-cylic acid . . . also known as aspirin. I know what you are saying: "Aspirin in my strawberries? No way!" But it is true. Salicylic acid is God's pesticide that the plant naturally produces, and some foods have higher concentrations of this chemical. Not so coincidentally, *all* the foods she was reacting to were at the *high* end of the salicylate list. And guess what else was on there. Almonds. They are very high in salicylates. So began experimental protocol #3,486—salicylate removal. Amazing result—increased speech, and lots of it. She had been acquiring speech all along, but the increased salicylate load seemed to somehow be blocking her from expressing it. Bye-bye, almond milk and almond flour, and hello, speech!

6. Salicylate intolerance and toxicity is very real and causes severe health issues (both physical and mental) for many children,

as well as adults. According to the Food Intolerance Network, "Research shows that about 20% of adults with asthma, 60% of people with food-induced itchy rashes, headaches or migraines, 70% of people with irritable bowel symptoms and 75% of children with behavior problems may be sensitive to salicylates."

Do you remember a condition called Reye's syndrome in the 1980s? This may be one of the most severe examples of salicylate sensitivity/toxicity. Children were becoming very ill, some dying, after taking aspirin during a viral illness like chicken pox or flu, leading to the warning on aspirin labels that aspirin was not recommended for children under nineteen. Epidemiological research has shown an association between the development of Reye's Syndrome and the use of aspirin (a salicylate compound). (Source: National Reyes Syndrome Foundation.)

Largely by trial and error and by consulting salicylate lists we found from researchers in Australia, we found thirty healthy, low-salicylate foods for our daughter. We started feeding her these, rotating them and trying to make them look and taste different so that she wouldn't lose interest in the diet that seemed to bring so much relief to so many of her symptoms. We have stuck to this diet, the "cave-baby" diet, as my husband refers to it, for the last three years, slowly trying to introduce new foods when she is stable and holding our breath that she does not react.

From our perspective, the diet and environmental changes along with avoiding chemicals she is sensitive to have taken significant burdens off her system. This has allowed her body to have peace and less pain. It has also allowed her brain to develop, and for her to grow physically, emotionally, and developmentally. We have now seen well over twenty specialists on our medical journey. This prestigious list includes four metabolic/mitochondrial specialists, who still can't agree on whether this is primary mitochondrial disease, despite the fact that hundreds of thousands of dollars of testing have been ordered, reported, and analyzed. She has remained in the "suspected mitochondrial disease" diagnostic category for the last three and a half years.

As time has worn on, we have become much less concerned about the formal diagnosis and the label. We are now much more focused on continuing to keep our daughter pain-free, growing, developing, healthy, and smiling more now than she ever did her first three years of life. Recently we consulted with a developmental pediatrician. He spent nearly two hours going through her medical history with a fine-tooth comb. At the end of the appointment, he said, "You did it, Mom." Confused, I said, "Did what?" He replied, "You saved her brain."

"I didn't do this, God did," I said.

"Okay, fair enough, but you listened," he concluded.

I trusted my gut, I researched, I made changes, I observed, I recorded my observations, I listened to that inner voice (which I truly believe was God's guidance). Our family witnessed my little girl retreat deep within herself, and we pulled with all our might to bring her back to our world. I have been blessed with a husband and family who support me, believe in my intuition, and help me do everything in our power to keep her here every day. By making changes to her diet and environment and by removing toxic insults to her system, we continue to see improvements—true improvements—and healing. After much searching we have found practitioners who truly "get it" and have helped us continue to help her. We still have rough days, but they are greatly outnumbered by the good ones. She is ready to enter kindergarten in a mainstream classroom. She is ice-skating, swimming, riding a bike, and having play dates with friends. She is prescription-medication-free (no more reflux roulette), and for us, these are all amazing accomplishments.

7. Mitochondrial disease can cause regressive autism and may be caused by a genetic defect, or triggered by environmental toxins, including (but not limited to): medications, anesthesia,

vaccines, and environmental exposures including pesticides. (For more information, see the following studies on pubmed.gov; they are listed here by their PubMed ID numbers: 16566887, 19043581, 25008905, 25883837, and 25956238.)

God really gets the last WINK on our journey. Without His eternal wisdom and guidance, the outcome would have been very different for our entire family. *John 8:32: And you will know the truth, and the truth will set you free.*

9

Co-Pilot
Fighting to Win

"Nothing can resist the human will that will stake even its existence on its stated purpose."

—Benjamin Disraeli

STANDING IN MY KITCHEN, I FEEL TUGGING ON THE BACK OF MY shirt. I turn around to see my five-year-old daughter, Emily, holding a Talk About Curing Autism magnet that says, "Autism is Treatable. Recovery is Happening." She asks me, "What does this say?" So I tell her. She looks down at the magnet and appears to be satisfied with the answer, so I go back to preparing dinner. She investigates further, "Mommy, what is autism?" I try my best to explain what autism is, and she tries to process my answer. I am delicate in my words. Such a sterile label for something so difficult. Nearly forbidden and spoken in hushed tones; always kept remote from Emily's name. Her next question was nothing I was prepared for.

"Mommy, do I have autism?"

I freeze.

How do I answer that? I thought it would be a while before we had this conversation. I'd always pictured her being a teenager when these questions came up (I have played out in my mind what questions she might have). And I was okay with that because she would be old enough to understand. We would have closure. The battle would be done. But here was my five-year-old standing at my side wanting answers now. Why was it so hard to give her an answer?

Truth is, I have spent too much time thinking about when would be a good time to talk about what she has been through and not enough time thinking about *what* I would say to her. Any time the thought enters my mind, it is quickly replaced with feelings of guilt. How do I tell her what happened to her? Will she blame me? Will she remember how hard we fought to help? I start thinking about the last five years and wonder how much she remembers.

Emily was born very early on a Wednesday morning. We are a military family, and at the time we were stationed in a small town in Oklahoma. I remember hearing the pelting rain and howling wind of the storm outside. But the moment she was born, I only felt peace in that room. I looked at her and saw a happy, healthy baby. I thought there was no way anything could go wrong. Life was so perfect. She was perfect.

For the first two months, everything was great. We did everything we were told. As first-time parents, who were we to question our pediatrician? Doctor's orders, right? That was until a family member gave us some information on vaccines and their potential harm. We were very confused. I had never had any reason to question vaccines. I was indoctrinated as a child into thinking that immunizations were important. As a parent, I was conditioned to think the same way.

During my daughter's two-month checkup, we asked questions about vaccines and their safety. Naively, we figured our pediatrician would be able to give us the pros and cons of vaccinating and would support our decision. Instead, he scolded us. So much for informed consent. By the end of the appointment, he had me convinced that my child would die of a disease if I didn't vaccinate. So I relented and Emily received the DTaP and HepB vaccines that day. A few hours later, she was cranky and had a fever, but by the next morning, those symptoms disappeared and she suddenly had reflux. We expressed our concerns to her doctor, but he spouted the CDC's dogma. He coldly declared our daughter fine.

A few months went by, and we went back in for more vaccines. At around seven months of age, it seemed like Emily had become weaker, and she was not sleeping well. But through the next several months, Emily continued to meet all her milestones. She loved to talk and learned new words quickly. She loved books and interacted with others. Her giggle and smile were enough to make anyone's day.

Military life demanded another move so we began seeing a new pediatrician. When Emily was nineteen months, we went in to get her the last DTaP and flu shot. Things were never the same after that; our daughter plateaued developmentally and stopped making expected gains. I made an appointment and expressed my concerns. Again, I was bullied and made to feel like a complete idiot. But this time, I wasn't going to let anyone convince us to do what we didn't feel was right. After a lengthy discussion, my husband and I decided to stop vaccinating Emily. We were too late. In the weeks following Emily's nineteen-month shots, her stomach became very distended. A few weeks after that, she was in the hospital for complications from the flu. While there, she received IV antibiotics. A few months later she got cellulitis (a bacterial skin infection). We still have no idea what caused it, but she was once again hospitalized and given IV antibiotics.

During this time, my husband was gone on his first deployment, so it was just Emily and I. Emily had never been very sick, so being hospitalized twice within a few months was puzzling. And it got worse. It seemed that every month there was something new.

Emily struggled with constipation for several weeks and then would switch to diarrhea. I made an appointment with her pediatrician. I was assured my daughter was merely struggling with her daddy being deployed. I left with a useless referral to a child psychologist. Absurd. I stood my ground and demanded a referral to a gastroenterologist. It took a few visits to make our case, but finally we had our referral. The gastroenterologist took some x-rays and performed a barium enema. The tests showed she was constipated, but everything else looked normal. They cleaned her out, but after a brief reprieve, the symptoms returned. I was worried but sought comfort in the test results. I continued to make excuses and find explanations for the things I was seeing. Then my wake-up call came.

When she was two, I enrolled Emily into a play-and-music class. I watched the other kids running around having fun and trying the activities, and I couldn't help but compare them to Emily. She stood close to my side with a look of panic and hands placed over her ears. She was so anxious that it took two months before she tried some of the activities. When she did, she couldn't do what the other kids were doing. She also showed no interest in the other kids; they seemed invisible to her. We eventually stopped going to the class as Emily began having anxiety any time we left the house. She spent most of the day crying and screaming, unable to communicate beyond the screams and pointing. When Emily wasn't screaming, she acted like a drunk. She would walk into walls, randomly fall over, and laugh hysterically for no reason.

Again, I found myself in the doctor's office airing my fears. I expected to leave with no answers, but that day was different. The pediatrician finally heard my concerns and referred her to be evaluated. I felt a bit relieved but also puzzled. I wanted answers, but I was also hoping to hear that my kid was okay, even though I knew she wasn't. I questioned the doctor as to what she felt was wrong. The answer was something I never thought I'd hear. "I want Emily to be evaluated for autism." *Autism?* That can't be. My world froze as I tried to process what I had just heard.

I looked down at my daughter, who was sitting on the floor anxiously pinching her neck. She had dark circles under her eyes and a look of pain on her face. Her stomach was huge, and I watched as she made uncomfortable swallows as she tried to keep the reflux down. My child was in physical pain. She was born happy and healthy, and then something changed. It didn't make sense. I began to wonder if the behavior and health concerns were connected, but her doctor assured me they weren't and would not offer any help for the pain. She felt that the physical symptoms I noticed were of no concern. This response bothered me. My child was visibly not well, but I was being told that she was fine.

I came home that day feeling so depressed. I sat at my computer for several hours reading about autism and trying to convince myself that Emily did not have that. But the more I read, the more I knew it was true. Two months later, she received a diagnosis of PDD-NOS. She was also delayed in fine motor skills, gross motor skills, and speech. She was very weak and had low muscle tone. Emily needed speech, occupational, physical, and feeding therapy.

When asked what things would look like in the long run, the doctor replied that our daughter would never function as a normal adult and there was not much hope of changing that. No hope? This couldn't be the answer. I knew it wasn't—there is always, always hope. Emily deserved better. I knew I had to fight for her. I was motivated to find answers and prove all of her doctors wrong.

At least I would not be fighting alone. My husband returned from his redeployment. I needed reinforcements. We turned to my husband's aunt, who had been through the same thing with her child. She pointed us in the right direction, and we started biomed. We owe everything to her and would not be where we are today without her help.

In addition to the help from our aunt, we got connected with Talk About Curing Autism, an organization that gave us access to a lot of helpful resources. Within a few weeks after Emily's diagnosis, we headed to our first appointment with an autism specialist. It was the first time I actually felt like we were getting somewhere. Within a few weeks, we had answers to so many of our concerns. We started with diet and added probiotics, melatonin, and vitamin B12 injections. After one week, some of the fog had lifted. The changes were noticeable, and we knew we were on the right track. Emily was talking more and was jubilant. It was major progress. But I could tell she was still having stomach problems.

Again, my husband's aunt came to the rescue and recommended a GI specialist in Texas who she was sure could help us. So we made the trip to Texas, and boy, was she right. After having Emily scoped, results showed her intestines were a total mess. It was hard to hear, but now we had more answers. We had more work to do.

Over the next several months, we worked with both our autism doctor and the GI specialist. The changes were amazing. Emily began communicating better. She began showing major improvements in physical therapy and conquering huge milestones we thought might never come. The reflux was finally gone, and for the first time Emily began eating meat. She had been on pureed food for the last year because she was too uncomfortable to eat regular food and did not have the strength to use utensils.

Emily continued to make giant leaps towards recovery. Her therapists were amazed as she met goal after goal and became more confident and less anxious. The transformation was amazing. I cried tears of joy with every victory, whether big or small. Every milestone was worth celebrating.

We were onto something, but despite seeing improvements, I wasn't ready to settle for "good enough." We had opened the door to recovery, and now that we knew it was possible, there was no looking back. I wanted answers to everything. We were still seeing a lot of progress, but with every leap forward, we would fall a few steps back. New things would pop up, and we would once again find ourselves confused and full of new questions.

When Emily was four years old, she got sick with a bad stomach flu, and for the first time in a long time we found ourselves in the hospital. She got through it, but shortly after that we began seeing bloating, stomach pain, sleeping problems, and some other odd symptoms. I found myself exhausted and needing inspiration to get out of this temporary setback.

Around that time, my husband bought me an amazing book, *The Thinking Moms' Revolution*. I read the book several times, feeling renewed hope. I was so inspired listening to the stories of moms who had been through the same thing and continued to fight for their kids. I knew I had to do the same. So we headed back to our doctor, did more testing, and a few weeks later Emily was doing better than ever.

Today, Emily is five years old and has lost her diagnosis. She is anxiety-free, her reflux is gone, her communication is great, her sensory problems have dissipated, and her physical strength has greatly improved. She is very happy and loves to socialize with others. We still deal with stomach problems from time to time, but I hold on to the hope that one day she will be permanently pain-free. We have come so far from where she was a few years ago, proving that anything is possible.

In survival training, the military teaches that a person can live three weeks without food, three days without water, three hours without shelter, three minutes without air, and only three seconds without hope. We never lost hope, and we kept fighting. There have been so many ups and downs in our journey to recovery. Looking back, it's hard not to feel guilt and sadness. But for the most part, I feel stronger than ever. I feel proud of my daughter. She should feel proud of herself. But the question still stands: Do I tell my daughter she has autism?

Emily is still standing in front of me, waiting for an answer. I can't put it off any longer. I choose my words carefully as to not cause too much confusion or frustration. "Emily, you were born very healthy and so happy. Then you got sick. So mommy and daddy worked really hard to help you, and you worked really hard to get stronger. Do you remember any of that?" She nods her head yes. I point back at the magnet, to the word *recovery*. "Recovery is happening!" I tell her in an excited voice. "Recovery means you are getting better and feeling healthy again. It means autism is gone. Do you feel better, Emily?" She thinks about it and pulls up her shirt to show me her belly. "Mommy, my tummy feels better. I feel happy." I smile at her. "That's all that matters, Emily. Recovery is all that matters." It's at that moment that the guilt over what happened is gone. Recovering her from this is all that matters. It's what we put our strength and energy into every day, and every day we are stronger for it. Does my daughter have autism? No, I can honestly tell her, she does not. Autism is gone. Recovery is happening!

10

Lioness
Trust Your Gut

"IF YOU WERE TO HEAR BAD NEWS, WOULD YOU WANT TO HEAR IT now or after you got some rest?" I was still in my postnatal, epidural-induced haze when my husband asked me this, so I did not "get" what he was telling me. I told him that I probably would want to hear the news before the nap, and then he told me they thought my newborn daughter had Down syndrome. The thought that he was joking briefly crossed my mind, but I knew this was something he wouldn't joke about.

You see, we had checked for this with a genetic counselor during an ultrasound in my twentieth week of pregnancy. It was the *big* thing that we were worried about. We had one "soft" marker for it, a calcium deposit on her heart. Then the counselor looked for her nasal bone. Apparently, the shortening or complete lack of it—I don't remember which—was a huge marker for DS, and we waited ten long agonizing minutes to find out if she had one.

My poor husband, being a true Sicilian and the only boy in a large family, wanted a boy of his own. Now he was discovering that not only was he having a girl, but he might also be having a child with Down syndrome. We both desperately wanted to find a nasal bone, and she finally allowed us to see it. Relieved, we went home with the comfort that our chance of having a child with Down syndrome was one in 145, not much. So we continued with this pregnancy, basking in the joy of having a healthy, "normal" baby on the way.

I continued to work at the local pet store and was planning to work until the middle of November, giving myself another four weeks to get ready for the baby, who was due in December. But I started to get very uncomfortable and left work earlier than intended. A few days later, I "sprung a leak," and the midwife induced me. At 11:19 p.m. on November 11, 2004, my sweet baby Mina was born, a little over three weeks early.

Mina was in the hospital NICU for six days, and she was hardly ever in my arms. I was having a hard time nursing due to all of the stress and the separation from her. She had been given IV antibiotics, probably because I had her the week before we were to do Group B strep testing. The treatment for a positive test is antibiotics, so they gave the antibiotics to her just in case. Even though she was a newborn, it took three nurses to hold her down to put in the IV. I think about this now and laugh because they had said that her "floppiness," among other things, led them to believe that she had DS. Even my sister-in-law remarked with astonishment that she couldn't be that weak and floppy if it took that many nurses to hold her down.

As many NICU moms know, there is always a flurry around the unit, and my child was one of those cooped up in what my husband has affectionately called the "baby spa," otherwise known as the bili lights, to treat jaundice. Finally, after six days of lights, CAT scans, IV antibiotics, and monitoring, they said she was ready to leave. We took our new family member home in an emotional blur. We were not even ready to have this baby yet—we had no furniture put together. And on top of it all, we had to take on something we had not been prepared for. We were bringing home a child with a disability, *the* disability we feared most.

When I worked at the pet store, I saw groups of older kids and adults with cognitive disabilities come in with their group home support and teachers. I always felt uncomfortable around these people. I feel ashamed to say this now. I felt like my boundaries were being invaded physically, as the people with Down syndrome tended to touch me or get right in my face to talk to me (and I couldn't always understand them). I think this reaction is what made me so upset about having a child with DS—that coupled with the way my mother impressed upon us that intelligence was extremely important, even more so than looks (not that people with Down syndrome aren't intelligent, but the common perception is that they are not.) At least that is what I picked up from her—she had never expressed that verbally. She even worked with people with disabilities as a nurse's aide, and her eyes would glow when she talked about the people she cared for. But, somehow, I picked up that in order to be worthwhile, I had to be the smartest person in the class. Or better yet, I should in my mind strive to be as perfect as I could be, matching the level of professional expertise of others in the areas of my interest. I had to *at least* be extremely intelligent. And here I was with a child who belonged to "that" group of people, and I wondered if I would ever be able to bond with her. My husband, God bless him, said to me, "Honey, if you can bond with a hamster, you can bond with her." That was all it took, and I knew then that I could let that thought go.

Time passed, and the fears started to melt away. Mina was such a cute baby, such a joy! Therapists came into the home through Early Intervention to work with her. We spent time getting to know our little girl and watched her blossom. Others used to comment on how bright her eyes were, how she seemed to be such a smart little thing. Meanwhile, my husband found Down syndrome support forums for me to join, so I made sure to do that. It was so nice to be connected to others who "got it."

Others were trying to help, too. One of my sisters and a sister-in-law found out about multivitamins for DS specifically, so with my dad's help, I bought some. I figured that with time, the therapies, and these vitamins, my daughter would become one of those "superstars" of DS that we heard about. She would be almost neurotypical, I was sure of it. I didn't want to accept the idea of her ending up as a bagger at a grocery store (I cringe at having even felt this way). She could do so much more.

When I brought her home, I tried to get her to nurse, but I wasn't producing much milk, and she was falling asleep at the breast. So after consulting a lactation specialist and failing miserably at our "assignment" to pump ten times and feed ten times each day for a couple of days, we decided to formula feed. This was a hard decision for me because in my eyes, each decision to not do the optimum for my child was a decision to not have her succeed.

Other than perhaps a little reflux, she did fine with the formula. She suffered from constipation, though, so our pediatrician had us use MiraLAX daily. Over a year or so, we were able to introduce baby foods to her—oatmeal cereal and some pureed meats. She was progressing well in terms of motor development and rolled all over the floor. She finally smiled and laughed, something that had seemed to be very slow to come, and that was so fun to see.

With the speech therapist, we eventually got her to chew some of the puffs and other mashable toddler foods. She loved Goldfish crackers and Cheerios. Those were her favorites! But in general, she wasn't a picky eater. The problem area for her was sleep. She would wake up crying at night and take half-hour naps. She began waking up for hours on end in the middle of the night. We had a sleep study done, but she wouldn't let the technicians put electrodes on her head. She was sensitive to people touching her head, particularly strangers bearing tape and wires, and she was also frightened. Though they weren't able to check brain wave patterns, they were able to determine that there was no apnea, so that was good, but there were no real answers to her sleep issues.

She did not seem to develop like the other children on the Down syndrome support forums, and she also didn't play with toys. I was told over and over by other moms that their children all developed at their own pace and in their own time. But this just didn't sit well with me, so one day, I decided to Google "child with Down syndrome doesn't play with toys." Nothing popped up for Down syndrome. However, a slew of articles came up that dealt with autism. So I decided to look at the diagnostic criteria, and what I saw shocked me. My daughter fit most of the traits of an autistic child! I told my husband, and then I consulted with all of her therapists. They all decided that she was too social to have autism; however, our developmental therapist agreed to contact our service coordinator to let her know our concerns.

We ended up having what was called a Medical Diagnostic Evaluation done, which involved a psychologist, a developmental pediatrician, and one other specialist. They interacted with Mina for three hours or so, and after doing so, told me that she was, in fact, too social to have autism, so her issues were chalked up to the delays caused by Down syndrome. We went home thinking that it was just a matter of time before she developed these skills. I returned to my forums determined to see what others did to help their children learn to play, and I was told many different things. Unfortunately, I had done all of these things, and nothing was working.

During this same period, we decided to have another child, and we figured that having a sibling would be great for Mina, too. I got pregnant with my youngest and gave birth to her in the fall of 2008.

During the infancy of my youngest, I found myself withdrawing more and more from the Down syndrome forums. It was too depressing seeing the difference between my child and the others. Mina was still not developing, and she seemed so reactive to any change in her environment. Every time we tried to take her somewhere and away from watching *Barney*, she would melt down. She refused most touch, and the light just seemed to have left her eyes. She hated getting her hair or body washed, and she only wanted to watch TV and eat copious amounts of crackers and Cheerios.

Meanwhile, my second child had issues sleeping, and I had to hold her during her naps. So, during those times, I read while she slept in my lap. I don't remember why, but I decided to read Jenny McCarthy's book *Healing and Preventing Autism*. I was dumbfounded to see that so many kids with autism had the same issues as my Mina, and I wondered if perhaps some of these things that worked for autism would help her. I also started to think that the evaluation that she'd had was incorrect, so I looked up the DSM IV and realized that Mina fit all of the diagnostic criteria for autism. I relayed my suspicions to our pediatrician, to her school social worker and psychologist, and to her therapists at Easter Seals.

The school psychologist said that after putting on her "autism" lenses, she began to see Mina's behaviors in a new light and noted what she discovered. The therapist at Easter Seals recommended presenting Mina to the Medical Advisory Board. We made three videos, one for each therapy session, and then presented the video to a board of physicians of different specialties to see what they recommended to us.

It was at this time that I began to give Mina probiotics and vitamin D. I also visited the nutritionist at Easter Seals, who recommended a high-dose multivitamin for malnourished children. Within a week of dosing Mina with the vitamin D, her therapists were talking about her eye contact and how it had improved. This was exciting news for me, and I knew I was onto something. The day before the MAB, we went to see a neurologist. After about thirty minutes of observing Mina jerking around and asking me questions, he said that she was, in fact, autistic. I felt an overwhelming sense of relief, but I wanted to be sure, so I waited to see what the MAB would have to say. The day came, and after it was over, the OT told me that after her three-minute-long video of Mina during her OT session, the developmental pediatrician said, "Before we go any further, you *do* realize this child has a secondary diagnosis of autism?" A-ha! I *knew* it! I felt vindicated. Finally! Answers and a direction to go in.

I read more about autism; I also started giving Mina her multivitamin. Mina's teacher, who had gone on maternity leave, came back and asked me who this new child was! I noticed it, too. It was like the world suddenly existed and she was seeing it for the first time. I decided that treating physical aspects of autism was really the way to go (and not therapies), so I took the money that would be going towards more therapy and directed it to her health instead.

We had a consult with Judy Converse, a dietician and nutritionist who herself has an autistic child, and we began the conversion to a gluten- and casein-free diet. All Mina ate was gluten- and casein-filled Gerber baby food, Cheerios, and Goldfish. This was going to be interesting. But after a little bit of sweat and cursing my existence, I was able to do it. Three days or so after removing the last bit of casein and gluten, she got a really high fever. I read about this reaction in Judy's book. Mina's body had stopped fighting food and was finally fighting "bugs!" After this fever was gone, she was smiling and laughing. Laughing! My daughter was laughing . . . and happy! And after a few months, she had lost about twelve pounds, pounds that she really needed to lose as she was getting heavy. I was really, really excited. And then I was really, really angry.

My daughter lost valuable time that she could have had to heal. Maybe she would have been chewing by now. We wasted time hearing that her big belly was just low tone. She wore an abdominal binder to support her back and gut. I know now that that bloating is from bacteria or yeast, as her belly only gets bigger at the end of the day after she has eaten. How uncomfortable that must have been. She should not have been fed crackers and cheese. They just made her sicker. Before she went gluten- and casein-free (and now grain-free), she had extremely low IgA levels in her stool test results. This indicated poor immune function, particularly in the gut. After a couple of years on the gluten-free, casein-free, and soy-free diet, we tested again, and the levels increased to the normal range.

She has been alert and is off multivitamins now because she is eating nutrient-dense food. I could have started earlier, and I cannot get that time back. I warn parents now to push for an evaluation if they suspect that their child with Down syndrome also has autism (one study has suggested that 18.2 percent of the DS population has autism.) I tell them to trust their guts and follow any and all information to get the resources they need to help their kids. I wish I could go back in time and do so for myself. I have apologized to Mina for not getting a second opinion, for not doing more sooner, and I am still working on forgiving myself and the professionals who should have known.

Since the diagnosis, we have tried supplements, dietary changes, and now homeopathy. Each change has brought gains, though Mina is one of those kids who responds slowly and steadily. She is not an overnight responder as many children with "just" autism are. She, like many other children with Down syndrome, takes more time to heal, doing it slowly and without spurts. She still doesn't talk, but she has gained sounds without losing them, has become engaged with her environment, and also handles changes in routine a little more easily. One of the best things to happen is that she cares that we exist. She has even cuddled, and that is HUGE for us! Just to be able to get a giggle or a snuggle out of her is priceless.

Up until this point, we have used some supplements, homeopathy, and are starting herbs now to heal her bloated belly. The biggest changes we have seen have been increases in cognition and flexibility. She is also much more "lovey dovey" these days and looks for her parents, sister, and even the cat, grabbing our faces in affection. Another factor that seems to be beneficial to her has been change in our attitude and viewpoint. The more open and accepting we are of her for who she is and where she is, the more she seems to respond to us.

Meanwhile, I am taking more time for myself and am trying to create a more loving and positive attitude in my home. The effects are astounding, and I wish I had let go of the stress sooner in the journey. I will follow what I think God is telling me to do, and then let go for the sake of Mina, for the sake of my family. I have a feeling that healing Mina will result in the healing of our family and ourselves. What started as a nightmare has become a blessing to my family. Would I have chosen this for us? No way! But God is using it to bring us to Him and to heal us all.

Some of you may be wondering what I think caused my daughter's autism. I have thought about it a lot. There is a much higher incidence of autism in the Down syndrome population than in the general population. Estimates run from 5 to 18.2 percent of the population, depending upon the source.[1] Some experts in the Down syndrome community have speculated that there is a genetic causation of the autism in Down syndrome. Some of us who are in the unique position of having a child with the dual diagnosis have other thoughts.

Personally, I think that people with Down syndrome have mitochondrial dysfunction. We all saw the news coverage of the Hannah Poling vaccine injury case. We know that she was suffering from undiagnosed mitochondrial dysfunction. It was ruled that this dysfunction was triggered by her vaccines, causing her to descend into autism. In people with Down syndrome, not only are there physical differences from neurotypical people (such as smaller nasal passageways and ear canals), but there are also physiological differences, which tend to be biochemical. One such difference is the insufficient production of glutathione, which is necessary for "taking out the

---

[1] See http://www.ncbi.nlm.nih.gov/pubmed/2035732.

trash," and detoxing heavy metals. There are other issues as well, like an increased chance of developing diabetes and leukemia.[2]

A lot of the choices I made as a parent clearly compromised my daughter, though I didn't know it at the time. I fully vaccinated her up until a certain age, even when a close family member expressed concern about vaccines and autism. But I did it anyway because the doctors all said that children with DS need to have all of the vaccines available because of their weak immune systems. I gave her MiraLAX to ease the constipation, a standard medication that is used by almost all children with Down syndrome. Mind you, this drug is now on the FDA watch list for neuropsychiatric events, under the name of polyethylene glycol. If you look at laxative labels, this drug is everywhere. I formula-fed her, gave her a high-gluten and dairy diet (celiac and sinus issues are frequent in Down syndrome), had a Terbutaline shot after I fell at work during the pregnancy, and had Pitocin, an epidural, and antibiotics during and after her birth. She also took antibiotics every time she had a sinus infection. All of these things contributed to her autism. I almost laugh when I hear people claiming that parents of kids with autism just want someone to blame, because ultimately I gave her autism. I made the poor choices that brought her to this place. So now I have had to do what I can to reverse the damage I caused by those choices.

As far as what I think needs to be done to reverse the downward spiral of our kids' health, it amounts to this: a massive overhaul of our environment, the food supply, the drug and chemical companies, and shutting down nuclear power. Our children's genes are being mutated, and their bodies are being destroyed by massive amounts of radiation. Then we feed them pseudo-food that is constantly being altered in the name of profit and supposed humanitarianism. Our children are sent to school as soon as possible and not given a proper

---

[2] This site offers more detail: dsdaytoday.blogspot.com/.

childhood, while parents are stressed out trying to feed their families. A whole societal overthrow needs to happen.

It starts with the choices we make as parents, and we can use this autism epidemic to wake people up. It is happening. I hear elderly people talk about skipping the doctor and taking Echinacea and vitamin C when they are sick. My own grandmother stopped getting the flu shot as she got sick every time she had one. Once she stopped, she stopped getting sick. We need to stand up as a people and demand change. We need to go back to "the good old days" of clean food, clean water, and community. We need to stop working so much and play more. Our kids' lives depend upon it.

11

Zorro
Crossing the Finish Line

T HERE WAS NO STARTING GUN TO MARK MY SON'S DESCENT INTO autism. There was no abrupt loss of skills or speech, no seizures or fevers, just an imperceptible braking until his forward momentum in life rolled to a stop somewhere between sixteen and twenty-two months.

I don't know if it was my own health—undiagnosed chronic Epstein-Barr and mycoplasma pneumonia—that set Connor up, or if it was my mouthful of leaky amalgams and fifteen years of mercury-filled flu shots. It could have been the case of Salmonella food poisoning that put me in the hospital for four days halfway through my pregnancy and stripped my GI tract.

Or it could have been the three ultrasounds I had, or the eighteen hours of Pitocin. Or was it the hepatitis B shot at birth? My son turned blue less than twenty-four hours later, but the doctor assured us that was a normal stress response. The MMR? Total vaccine load? After every well-child appointment, I had to clear my calendar for a week, because I knew I'd have an extremely fussy and feverish baby who would nurse constantly.

Whatever it was that lowered my boy's resistance and increased his risk, I'll never know with complete certainty.

What I do know is that by the time he was twenty-two months old, my beautiful boy was speaking less and less, having peaked at sixteen months with the phrase "Too hot to eat the pizza!" His anxiety increased daily. He would fall apart at loud noises, throw epic tantrums over nothing, and howl with fright if something startled him. Changes in routine, even throwing in one extra errand, triggered screaming fits. To the outside world, it probably looked like he was a spoiled brat who exploded over nothing. We couldn't leave the house without several pacifiers—one in his mouth and one in each hand—and his blanket that he wrapped around his head. And yet, three pediatricians in three states assured me that he was fine.

He was not fine. I was not fine. I took on a full load of guilt—the guilt I produced myself and the guilt lobbed at me by other people. There was something off about my kid, so as the mom, it was clearly my fault. I was reminded of this failing daily, from evil stares when I tried to contain monumental meltdowns while shopping or at the library, to helpful strangers suggesting my son would be fine if I just took a strap to him now and then, to flat out assessments that I was a terrible mother and this was *all my fault*.

The summer of 2001 leading up to our son's diagnosis was particularly hard. He wouldn't let me get a toothbrush in his mouth to brush his teeth, so he needed to have two stainless steel caps and four amalgam fillings put in while he was under sedation. When he came out of it, he howled for a solid hour. Howled like a wounded wolf. It was hideous.

A few weeks later, he fell and banged up his knees so badly he refused to walk for nine weeks. The pediatric orthopedic specialist thought he must have bruised the *inside* of the patella. No one could figure out why he wasn't walking, and we didn't know if he'd ever try again. Our best guess for his refusal to walk was that it simply hurt too much. It was just one more incident in a string of mysterious and unexpected behaviors. It took weeks before he was willing to try again, and by that time he'd lost a lot of muscle mass in his little legs.

We were drowning. Every day was a struggle, and we didn't know why. Our pediatrician waited until my son was three to agree that it might be time for a speech evaluation. I didn't know that I could seek that out on my own. It took six months to get an appointment. By then, I had to wheel Connor in the stroller to the desk because he couldn't or wouldn't walk.

The speech therapist said that, in addition to pronounced echolalia and expressive speech in the 2nd percentile, our son had cognitive delays, and we should get an evaluation. Looking back, I realized that she knew what was going on immediately, but couldn't say it because she wasn't qualified by the state to diagnose autism officially. We found a special preschool class for children with speech delays and got a referral for a complete neuropsychological evaluation. Then September 11, 2001, happened, and everything shut down, including our scheduled intake appointment.

One night in the midst of the multi-day assessment, I broke down crying after I'd put Connor to bed. My thoughts were reduced to a sobbing prayer of "Help us, please, help us." A very calm and clear message interrupted my sobs, almost like someone was speaking to me, and said, "Jill, everything's going to be alright." I stopped cold. There have been two occasions in my life when I heard this tiny, powerful voice. This was the first. It raised my spirits enough that the rest of the process didn't overwhelm me as much as it could have, but it rendered me defenseless for the actual diagnosis. I thought everything was going to be okay, and suddenly the floor caved in under me.

Honestly, any autism mom could have taken one look at Connor gripping a Thomas train in one hand and lining up rocks with the other at age two and a half and given me the answer, but due diligence must be done, the piper paid, et cetera. And so, autism: a full 299.0 diagnosis, not some lesser PDD-NOS (Pervasive Developmental Delay-Not Otherwise Specified) or even Asperger's. Connor had some speech, but it was almost exclusively echolalia—meaningless repetition. He ran in circles, jumped up and down for hours, flapped his hands, walked on his toes, lined things up, tantrumed, and flipped out if I took an alternate route while driving. He also had no friends, and he never made eye contact.

Dr. B., the psychologist who did the full neuro-developmental assessment, which examined everything from socialization and psychological maturity to academics, stopped after she made the pronouncement. "Mrs. R, are you breathing?" Not so much. I only remember snippets from that appointment, the highlights being:

1) My son would probably never make friends on his own;
2) We could take comfort in the fact that he wasn't technically mentally retarded because his IQ was above 70;
3) He was too inflexible and anxious for applied behavioral analysis therapy; and
4) We shouldn't be asking questions about whether he'll go to college, have friends, or get married.

We were gobsmacked. Autism was something at the periphery of my awareness, something that happened to other people, but only rarely. They couldn't mean my boy—he was so affectionate. Autism meant cold and unattached, unwilling or unable to display affection, right? What was autism? What was going to happen to my son? What could we do? Based on our previous experience with a scary diagnosis (my father-in-law's cancer), I knew my mother-in-law would ask about dietary changes, so we asked Dr. B. about that. She kind of brushed that aside, mumbling something about how there have been no double-blind, placebo-controlled studies, and directed us to the family resource room at the clinic. We dutifully listened, then headed home in a daze. I think I was able to talk about the diagnosis for about twelve hours before the shock and adrenaline wore off and the sadness that comes in the wake of a diagnosis took over, but it was long enough to make a couple of phone calls to our families and a couple of friends.

I'm a die-hard bookworm, and I come from a long line of readers. My first step in the direction of *doing something* was to head to the bookstore. I cleaned them out of books on autism. In 2001, that meant I got five books. My mom, who was 2,500 miles away, found one book: *Unraveling the Mystery of Autism and Pervasive Developmental Disorder* by Karyn Seroussi. That was the only book on the shelf at Books-A-Million in Goodlettsville, Tennessee, so that was the one my mom bought. I had the same book in my stack, but it was at the bottom.

Two days later, my mom called me, likely in tears, because we were all a sobbing mess, and told me to put down whatever I was doing and read that book. Now! So I did. That changed everything. That book saved my son. It gave me the information I needed to make a difference in his health and set us on a healing path. It also gave me something to *do*, which was in some ways more important for my ability to cope in light of my overwhelming feeling of helplessness.

Unraveling focused on one family's success with a gluten-free and casein-free (wheat- and dairy-free) diet. My husband wasn't keen to change our son's diet. Connor was living on bagels and chocolate milk. I could see his point—how could we take away the only two food groups Connor was eating?—but I had grabbed onto a shred of hope, and I wasn't letting go. I didn't care if it was hard. I was willing to crawl through glass for a 1 percent improvement. That book gave me hope, but more importantly, it gave me direction. I took milk out of my son's diet the next day. My niece Chloe had a milk allergy, so I already had some organic soy milk in the house. (Gluten would present a thornier challenge.)

Working on the assumption that it is easier to ask forgiveness than permission, I changed Connor's diet when my husband was on a weeklong trip out of town. I started by taking out milk. Within two days, he stopped running in circles. Within two weeks, he had adopted his cousin's stuffed bunny, renamed him Carrots, and started singing lullabies to him and pretending to put him to bed. This was his first pretend play, his first symbolic interaction with a toy. That bullet point of the diagnosis code—the notable absence of pretend play—was crumbling away. There was no way I was giving that bunny back. Sorry, Chloe. My husband read *Unraveling* on his next plane trip and came home ready to dive into a fully gluten-free/casein-free diet. Good thing I'd already started. And so we were off.

I found a small group of parents who had started a local biomed support group. Those parents became a lifeline. They connected me to doctors and therapists, pointed me to online support and resources, and became my friends. A few months in, I was more determined than ever to go further down the rabbit hole of alternative treatments in pursuit of better health. We found a Defeat Autism Now! doctor out of state who was a godsend, Dr. John Green in Oregon City, Oregon. He was our team leader and a true thought partner. He helped us save our son, and he is a wonderful human being who has compassion, who listens, and who thinks outside the box. (We love you, Dr. Green!) Our mainstream pediatrician, on the other hand, fired us from his practice for asking questions. I'd taken Connor in for a bump on the head and got a lecture about keeping up with the MMR. *Why?* I asked. And then I was told by the office manager to never darken their door again.

Our first order of business was to safely replace the amalgams in Connor's mouth with composite fillings, ramp up his mineral intake, and get chelation going. The connection between mercury and autism was compelling enough to us to pursue something called chelation, the removal of heavy metals through medicine that would literally grab the metals and carry them out of the body. This would include any lead that could have been lurking in his body as well—we had lived in an old house for a few years when he was born and knew that lead paint was present on the property. We needed to address heavy metal toxins, and our doctor wasn't going to proceed if Connor had a mouthful of silver (read: mercury) amalgams. I'm not sure if it was the action of removing mercury, the powerful antioxidant properties of the DMPS, the chelating medicine Connor's doctor prescribed, or the giant bolus of sulphur it delivers, but Connor did beautifully with the first round of oral chelation. His mood leveled out, he slept well, and he was more connected and interactive with the world around him

The school week following our first chelating weekend was interesting. Two of the most skeptical therapists we had—top-notch speech therapists that had zero faith in biomed and special diets—both came to me to tell me Connor had turned a corner and they had seen significant improvement just that week. He was expressing a newfound sense of humor and was participating more in the group. I mentioned to the first therapist that I suspected the new treatment we started was helping. She just rolled her eyes. When the second therapist mentioned the slew of emerging skills, I just smiled.

We became early adopters of biomedical interventions. We tried chelation, IVs, targeted nutrition, antifungals, antibiotics, methyl B12, and supplements. I attended conferences. I read books, medical papers, and online information. I took classes and even got through half of a degree in naturopathy before the school closed down. I was obsessed with helping my son improve. There were many problems to overcome. He had eczema, a million food allergies, sky-high antibody counts, or viral titers—especially for measles, intractable yeast and clostridia overgrowth, heavy metals, oxidative stress, nutritional deficiencies, low-level mitochondrial dysfunction, chronic diarrhea, bowel impactions, reflux, leaky gut, plus weak nails and brittle hair. For a year or two he didn't gain any weight, and his sleep—which had always been good—went to hell when he was five. We tested everything for signs of nutritional imbalance, immune dysregulation, toxin load, and other health markers: hair, pee, poop, blood.

As we addressed the health issues that all the testing uncovered, Connor's behavior, language, and connection with the world improved. Recovery from autism wasn't even a concept I entertained. We just needed to help him be as healthy as possible. If day-to-day life got better for us all, so much the better. I couldn't think more than three months ahead until our next doctor's appointment. It was an immediate and narrowly focused life, but it paid off. My son began to emerge from the fog of pain and disconnection. He gained three years of expressive speech in twelve months. He stopped tantruming. Life got easier for everyone, and I had a fire in my belly.

By the time Connor was six, we were able to start thinking about that second baby we'd always planned on. We chose adoption, and we brought our son Kyle home just before Connor turned seven. (The second time I heard that tiny, powerful voice was when I took Kyle's birth mom to the doctor just before Kyle was born and heard his heartbeat on the Doppler. I had an overwhelming jolt of recognition: "That's my boy!") By then, I was starting to consider the possibility of recovery. When Connor was in second grade, we had him reevaluated. The psychologist didn't remove the diagnosis, but downgraded him to "very mild PDD." He also registered a nearly 50-point improvement in his IQ scores.

It was interesting to me that none of the psychologists or educational therapists involved in that reevaluation asked us what we were doing to help our son, as if that kind of overall improvement and increase in IQ scores happens every day.

Connor's recovery wasn't fast, cheap, or easy, however. He had several plateaus and at least two significant and scary regressions. There would be weeks of no improvement. The regressions were the worst, stretches of time where all the gains he'd made in language acquisition would evaporate and his behavior would deteriorate with increased tantrums and decreased flexibility. I'm not sure what triggered the first one, but the second, and more significant, came in the wake of being exposed to toxic fumes during construction at his school. He went from being a connected, with-it kid back to the boy who didn't talk and who spent hours a day lying on his stomach rolling the Thomas train back and forth just inches from his nose.

Those two regressions showed me there was definitely something biological going on. With the right support—whether it was changing his supplements, addressing allergies, or pulling him from a toxin-filled environment—all his previous gains would return, sometimes in fits and starts, but they returned. He made another huge leap in improvement after age nine when we added an extensive regimen of combination homeopathy under the direction of our holistic pediatrician. (We love you, Dr. Elisa Song!) Every morning and evening I would mix his prescribed dose of up to ten different remedies—five drops of one, ten of another, thirty of a third—feeling like a mad scientist but seeing definite improvement across the board. We prepped him for another round of prescription antifungals, and the combination of the two approaches clinched it. We've never had to look at that kind of treatment since. His gut appears to have been healed to the point that his own immune system could take over and maintain that same level of health.

Today Connor is eighteen and he has recovered from autism. He had a few bumpy years with depression and anxiety when he hit puberty (*do not* underestimate puberty), but he has come out the other side with the help of excellent medical and therapeutic care. When he was sixteen, we ran a series of tests like we used to do when we first started treating him. Everything looked great: the number and severity of food allergies has decreased dramatically, and all the metabolic markers were normal. The test results for organic acids, dysbiosis, and gut function were all pretty much perfect. I got teary looking at them, and I swear I'd frame them if it wouldn't mortify him.

Around this time, Connor decided he wanted to get ripped. He changed his diet, adopting a primal approach. He also started working out intensely, starting with the weight room at school and some T25 DVDs. He shed more than 40 pounds and, yes, he got ripped. The best part of this transformation is that the anxiety and depression that had stalked him for years simply evaporated.

He is a lovely young man: kind, good-natured, and good-humored. He loves movies, heavy metal, and theater. He takes a stand on the side of social justice in all things and thinks about life and the people he encounters. He was awarded both Junior of the Year and Senior of the Year by the faculty at his high school, he has his driver's license, and he's off to a great college in the fall to study mathematics and philosophy. I couldn't be happier or prouder. And he is happy that when he's out with friends, he can have the occasional pizza with no ill effect. (Yes, a whole pizza. Teen boys and their appetites.)

So what did we do to get here? A fairly complete list includes: gluten-free/casein-free diet, removal of all allergens, antioxidants, high-dose vitamin A, herbs, homeopathy (both classical and combination), antibiotics, antifungals, enzymes, probiotics, methyl B12, TMG, folinic acid, DMPS chelation (both oral and transdermal), N-acetyl cysteine transdermal lotion, TTFD, glutathione (both IV and transdermal), craniosacral therapy, BodyTalk, and lots of prayer from every corner.

Keep in mind that the above was in addition to occupational therapy with sensory integration two to four times per week, Special Ed preschool, full inclusion through second grade, speech therapy, social skills groups, Floortime, RDI, special needs soccer, and karate.

Some things we tried didn't work or caused a negative reaction. I had a very sensitive kid and had to go very slowly. For example, I tried eight different enzymes before I hit on one that worked. I begged for samples from my support group and went through them one at a time. One gave Connor stomachaches, another gave him an eczema flare, and a third triggered odd behavior. Vitamin B6 was pretty much a disaster. I never completely understood why, but it took six years of healing before we were able to introduce it in a very small dose in the P5P form.

Food allergies and his extreme pickiness limited his diet. A trial of the Specific Carbohydrate Diet exacerbated his eczema and food allergies, so we went back to what had worked before. Please note: I recovered my kid during a six-year period where he never ate more than eight different foods—usually chicken nuggets, French fries, meatballs, muffins, fruit smoothies, rice, and potato chips. Kids with autism can be outrageously picky eaters. Whether it's a sensory issue, where they don't like the way the food feels in their mouths, or anxiety about something different, it can be a real challenge to get some of them to eat more than a handful of different foods. My son was one of those extremely picky kids. My point? Please don't allow a kid's limited menu to dissuade any attempts at a healing diet.

Yes, we were lucky. My son responded early and consistently enough to show me that there was a definite biological basis to his autism. But it wasn't just luck; we didn't give up when we got overwhelmed. I was devoted to his recovery to the exclusion of just about everything else. If something didn't work or he hit a plateau, I just maintained until I had enough energy or found a new approach to the issue and pushed forward. There was always something new on the horizon and always, *always* there was hope. In the end, that still, powerful voice was right: everything is all right. It just took a lot more time and effort than I ever could have imagined to cross that finish line.

I was also lucky—and I'm still lucky—that my husband stood shoulder-to-shoulder with me on this. We never stopped moving forward. No matter how dark my own world was (at one point, I couldn't drive my son to therapy without having a panic attack myself) or how expensive the treatments were, we didn't stop. It was worth it. Hope is always worth it.

So, what have I learned? What wisdom can I impart?

1.   The child is the gift. Autism? Not so much.
2.   There's always room for improvement.
3.   You haven't tried everything. Catch your breath, dive in again.

4. You're not alone.
5. Take care of yourself, because you're the engine that runs the show.
6. Find a way to forgive.
7. The body, the brain, the behavior—it's all connected.
8. Your health, your child's progress, the quality of your food, the toxicity of the environment—it's all connected.
9. Love your child at every step. Meet them where they are.
10. Strive to come from a place of LOVE.

12

Frankie
Recovery Is a Winding Road

"What lies behind us and what lies before us are tiny matters compared to what lies within us."

—Ralph Waldo Emerson

"Is the game on yet, Dad?" my son, Josh, yells from the top of the stairs.

"Almost. You've got ten minutes till it starts."

"Okay. I'll get my Seahawks shirt on."

This has been a regular exchange at my house during football Sundays this year. It's not that my ten-year-old son loves football, or any sport for that matter really—except for swimming; he would definitely choose to live in the water if we let him—but he knows how important the game is to his dad, and he's been putting forth an effort to connect with him on what he's interested in.

Football Sunday used to be my errand-running day, but now I prefer to stay at home and watch the game. It's not that I'm a diehard fan, either. The best part for me is watching my son engage his dad over football. It's a common theme across America, fathers and sons bonding over their mutual passion for a sports team. Most people don't even think about it; it's just a given. But when you have a child affected by autism, one thing you know with all your heart is that there are no givens. Everything is painstakingly worked for.

Josh has come so far since he was diagnosed at age three with PDD-NOS (Pervasive Developmental Delay-Not Otherwise Specified). At the time, he was stuck in his own world of spinning, throwing tantrums, dragging his head on the floor, and lining up his toys. He didn't communicate verbally, unless you count the screaming, and was constantly plagued by diarrhea.

The specialists we looked to for answers and solutions told us he would only progress minimally with traditional therapies (i.e., speech and behavioral therapy). They stressed that the best thing we could do for him, for us, was to accept this fact and begin planning his future. They, the experts, recommended looking into group homes, state-run facilities, or other living arrangements for him when he reached adulthood. They told us not to waste our money or place hope on the promises of alternative medicine doctors—they were snake oil salesmen preying on desperate parents. The gluten- and casein-free diet? Dangerous. Supplements? Ineffective. Postponing vaccinations? Deadly.

Well, the experts were right about one thing: Josh was only progressing minimally with traditional therapies. Not because they are ineffective, but because Josh would only participate for a half-second during his therapy sessions. The biggest success we had during these sessions was getting him to sit without him screaming, hitting, or head-butting us. The rest of the time was spent corralling him as he ran around the room like a madman, throwing tantrums (or his juice cup) because the therapist was trying to get him to do activities he didn't want to do. I knew there had to be more we could do to help him.

It's a very scary place to be, when your child is suffering and the people that should help actually don't, won't, or can't. After spending nine months post-diagnosis seeking help from doctors to no avail, we accepted the fact that our son's health and future were completely in our hands. It was time to get to work. I got my Google on, searching for alternative treatments for autism. My search led me to the Generation Rescue website, only weeks after it had gone online. That's where I read the words that would change the course of my son's life: AUTISM IS REVERSIBLE.

I had opened the information floodgates and spent every hour I could keep my eyes open taking it all in. Endless articles, studies, and parent testimonials discussing the role of environmental toxins and how changing the diet and addressing underlying medical issues can lessen symptoms of autism and even reverse them completely. These were things I had never been told by the medical doctors we had seen. The Autism Research Institute's website was a valuable guide. I wish TMR (Thinking Moms' Revolution) and TACA (Talk About Curing Autism) had been around at that time, as I think they are amazing sources of knowledge, hope, and support. Kenneth Bock's *Healing the New Childhood Epidemics* helped me a lot as well.

Being a military family and living in a small town did not leave us many options for alternative care. The closest doctor that practiced what used to be called the Defeat Autism Now! (DAN!) protocols was five hours away and had a year-long waitlist. Not wanting to waste any more time, I developed a plan, based on the various books and websites I had immersed myself in, of things I could do on my own to reverse Josh's autism. With my husband on board, we began implementing my plan.

We started the gluten- and casein-free diet and saw our son's behavior transform. We also saw his very first solid bowel movement. When you have a child who has only had diarrhea their entire four years of life, this is a very big deal. I was tempted to dip that log in gold and mount it on the wall! The tantrums were noticeably decreasing. He was looking into our eyes and connecting with us more. His therapists noticed a big change in how he was participating in his sessions. All of this happened within just two weeks of changing his diet. Yep, the very diet we were told was "dangerous" was bringing our son out of the pain he had been in since birth. His severe colic early in life was always chalked up to being "one of those things some babies have." Now I understood that his body had been under severe distress. He was hurting, and the only way to communicate that was by screaming.

After seeing the changes the diet had brought about in Josh, we started implementing the rest of the plan I had drawn out. We used magnesium salt baths to detoxify his body, and we removed all toxic cleaners and other products from the house. We started giving him the SuperNuThera vitamin supplement, MB12 nasal spray, and probiotics. All of these things led to improvements in Josh's behavior, his ability to focus, and his language development.

Some of the information I had come across online mentioned the possibility that vaccines were a trigger for autism for some children. I read many parent testimonials that stated their child's autism symptoms began abruptly after receiving vaccines. I read so many stories of children who were developing normally, had a round of shots, and in a matter of days developed autism. After reading that information, even though Josh had never had a noticeable regression after vaccination, I decided to put Josh's vaccines on hold until I could look further into the idea. In hindsight, his high-pitched screaming, arching of the back, and fevers following vaccination were reaction red flags, signs his immune system was overwhelmed, but I didn't connect this or his early issues of severe colic and not reaching milestones in infancy as being caused by his vaccinations at the time. His development had been delayed from the start, most likely from the flu shot, multiple doses of RhoGAM, antibiotics, and heartburn medication I received during my pregnancy with him. In that sense, his story was unlike those of children who were walking, talking and happy and lost all of those skills directly following vaccination. Every specialist we saw said it was proven that there wasn't any link, and what did I know, I was just a mom, not a doctor (yes, I would love to go back and smack myself in the face).

Life was moving forward. After spending six years in the military, my husband decided it was time to move on and create a more stable home environment for Josh. We relocated to California, where there were more resources for children with autism. We were beginning to let ourselves feel hopeful and optimistic about the future that was unfolding for Josh and our family.

It's amazing how life can change in an instant. This moment happened in our new pediatrician's office as Josh was getting his physical to enroll in school. The doctor took one look at his vaccination records and went into attack mode: "Do you know you are putting your son at risk of death?! This is the most irresponsible thing you could do as a parent! If you walk out of here without getting some of these vaccines, and he contracts an illness and dies, how are you going to live with that for the rest of your life?!"

Cue the inner doubt dialogue: *What if I am putting him at serious risk? Maybe just one, as long as it's not the MMR. That's the only one being questioned as a link to autism anyway. Josh never had a sudden regression after his shots in the past. Just one. Then I'll know I'm not putting his life in danger.*

It only takes a few seconds to make an irrational decision based on fear. This was one of those moments, and it is now one of the biggest regrets of my life. I left the office in tears, knowing I had made a serious mistake allowing Josh to receive the DTaP vaccine. Within forty-eight hours, Josh started losing the gains he had made over the last year and a half. Words disappeared and were replaced with crying, his eye contact decreased, and he started withdrawing into his own little world again. I don't know if I will ever be able to forgive myself. I try not to think about it too often because when I do, it takes me to a dark place, and when you are trying to save your child, you don't have time for dark places.

I immediately went back to the Generation Rescue website and contacted one of their Rescue Angels (parents of children with autism who volunteer to mentor other parents looking for local resources and doctor recommendations) for a referral to a DAN! doctor. My intervention plan had been child's play, and I now needed the big guns to undo the damage of the DTaP vaccine. I was referred to Dr. Karima Hirani near Santa Monica. It's hard to put into words the feeling of finding a medical professional who understands and truly listens to you and doesn't dismiss your concerns. It was such a relief to finally have a doctor in our corner who could, would, and did help us. We started the Valtrax/Nystatin protocol, IgG and IgE for food allergies, vitamins, minerals, amino acids, and MB12 injections, and within a few months, we were able to bring Josh back to baseline (where he was developmentally before the DTaP shot). Dr. Hirani had suggested chelation after getting lab results back—Josh's aluminum and arsenic levels were high—but I wasn't comfortable with it. From what little I had read about chelation, I thought it was too aggressive and too hard on the body. There are different forms of chelation, but the main objective of chelating agents is to remove heavy metals from the body.

Over the next six months, Josh continued to slowly progress from baseline, but eventually seemed to be hitting a plateau. After revisiting the research on chelation, I decided it was the right time to try the protocol. Josh's vitamin and mineral levels were looking good. Chelation can be hard on the liver, so it's very important that liver function be monitored throughout the process. Dr. Hirani assured me that his liver was healthy and able to handle it and that she would closely monitor the situation.

My motivation with trying interventions for Josh has always been the fact that I don't want to look back ten years from now and say I wish we would've tried it. That's not to say I am willing to try everything, but if I feel there is little risk and the effectiveness has been shown, and I feel it is a good fit for Josh, then I climb on board.

After a provocation test to determine which chelating agent worked best in his body, we moved forward with DMPS chelation. We chose to do the suppository version because it is less demanding on the body than having the chelating agents administered intravenously, and it's more effective than the oral or transdermal method. Two weeks after starting the treatment, I got a call from Josh's teacher asking me what we were doing with Josh. As with any treatment we've done, I refrain from informing his teachers/therapists of what we are doing so we can have an unbiased opinion. I told her I didn't want to say anything yet. "Well, whatever you're doing is working. Josh has a surprise to show you when he gets home!" his teacher told me.

Josh got home from school, walked through the door, and said, "I want paper and pencil." Whoa! He had *never* used the phrase "I want" before. This was huge! I happily obliged and figured he was going to scribble as usual. What I didn't expect was to look down and see him writing the *entire* alphabet! This child, who had fought me so hard on hand-over-hand tracing the letters of his name, who had made me write the alphabet on the chalkboard in his room ten times every night but would scream if I even tried to put the chalk close to his hand, was now writing all the letters. He showed me his finished work and, with a huge grin, said, "Alphabet letters." Then he asked for more paper, at which time I handed him the entire stack of printer paper. He wrote the letters out again and this time added his name and the numbers one through fifteen. I called my husband at work and asked him to come home. I was scared it was just temporary, and I wanted to make sure my husband got to experience it. Well, he did, and we were both puddles on the floor.

The next morning, our oldest daughter came running into our room. "Mom! Dad! Did you guys write words on Josh's chalkboard?" Still half-asleep, my husband and I opened the door to Josh's room to see him standing in front of his chalkboard, chalk in hand, and the words "BOX" and "FOX" written on the board.

"Josh? Did you write those words?" I asked him.

"Yes—box, fox," he replied, with the largest grin on his face.

In total disbelief, I asked him if he could write some more. He turned to the chalkboard and wrote "MOM" and "DAD." I looked at my husband, mouth hanging open. We both had tears rolling down our faces. He said, "We are going to Disneyland today." And that's just what we did.

Josh continued to make progress in leaps and bounds. We tried a couple more rounds of chelation, once intravenously, but never saw the huge spike in improvement like we had the first time. Josh was enrolled in the autism program at school but had improved enough to spend part of the day in a regular classroom during his kindergarten year and also in first grade. He was always ahead academically, but socially, emotionally, and behaviorally, he lagged behind his peers. He had a difficult time interacting with other children and struggled with back and forth conversation. He had a hard time calming himself down when he was angry or frustrated, which would cause disruptions in class.

In second grade, Josh was mainstreamed full time. There were a few bumps, but he continued to make progress mainly because his teacher had previously taught in special education classrooms and was experienced in handling kids who needed extra involvement. Third grade proved to be more difficult, as he was no longer ahead of his peers academically, and in turn, his behavior became more erratic. I was constantly getting calls from the school informing me of his classroom outbursts or refusal to participate in class. Kids were beginning to bully him daily. I had always thought that if Josh could get to the point where he was fully mainstreamed, autism would be behind us for good. I've since learned that recovery, for us, is an evolving journey. Some people cross that finish line with their child and no longer need any supports in place to maintain recovery. I hope to one day reach that place with Josh, but for now, although he no longer fulfills the clinical guidelines for an autism diagnosis, there are some lingering issues that make life a little harder for him. We continue to try and help his body, mind, and spirit heal.

The most recent treatment we've tried is called rTMS (repetitive Transcranial Magnetic Stimulation) being done by the Brain Treatment Center in Irvine, California. It's a technology that has been around for some time, mainly used as treatment for depression, seizures, and psychiatric disorders, but it is also showing promise in helping people with autism. The treatments consist of gently pulsing certain areas of the brain with an electromagnetic device to speed up or slow down brainwaves. It can stimulate areas of the brain, specifically neurons that aren't firing like they should be.

We decided to have Josh partake in the trial to see if he was a viable candidate for treatment. It was a weeklong process, and on the first day, Josh's EEG indicated a lack of activity in the frontal lobe and his brainwaves were not in sync. These test results garnered him a go-ahead on the treatment. Dr. Jin and his team were caring, insightful, and a goldmine of information. That alone made this treatment worth it for us. We ended the week with a second EEG to see if the rTMS was working well enough to justify continuing treatment. We, as well as the team, were surprised by the results—Josh's brain had responded so well to just four sessions that he was no longer a candidate for treatment based on the changes in his brainwaves, and also his brain activity had increased significantly in the frontal lobe, an area of the brain that lacks activity in many people with autism. It's responsible for emotions, behavior, speech, and abstract reasoning – things many children on the spectrum struggle with. We saw improvements in all of these areas immediately following treatment and continuous improvements months after treatment.

Looking back on our journey of recovery with Josh, we've experienced many moments I thought would never happen because his doctors told us they wouldn't. From hearing him say "I love you," to competing on the school's swim team and now sitting with his dad enthusiastically watching the football game, these moments are never taken for granted. It pains me to think that had we listened to the doctors and given up hope, we might not have ever gotten to know Josh like we do now. He has a big heart and a sharp sense of humor, and he keeps us on our toes. He has taught us to appreciate the little things, to enjoy the good times, to be patient during the bumps in the road, and no matter what, to keep going and keep fighting.

Update

Since writing this chapter, I decided to homeschool Josh, and it has made a major difference in his behavior and anxiety levels. I really wish I had done it sooner! Any issues we were still dealing with have pretty much disappeared. We did see some behavioral regression with the onset of puberty—he became aggressive, less engaged, easily angered, and difficult to reason with (I'm really looking forward to the TMR book on puberty coming out in Fall 2016!). For now, we seem to have found the right supports to keep him even keeled.

Josh has also been diagnosed with Lyme disease. I have learned that many children on the spectrum, and in fact a large percentage of the population in general, have underlying Lyme. I urge you to look into this for your child, as many Lyme symptoms present similarly to autism symptoms in our children. I suggest watching some of Dr. Klinghardt's videos on YouTube. He is one of the most well-versed Lyme doctors out there, and I have gained great insight by hearing him speak at conferences and through his videos.

So many people have had a hand in helping Josh overcome the obstacles he has been faced with. Our family, my Team TMR/TMR family, so many amazing autism parents I've met in person or on Facebook over the years, and the practitioners who work alongside us all . . . Thank you, from the bottom of our hearts, for helping and supporting us through this journey. I'm forever grateful.

13

Green Bean Girl
No Excuses—You Can Change Your Child's Life

"WHAT I WAS REALLY HOPING TO HEAR ABOUT WAS YOUR EXPERIENCES after HBOT and the chiropractor." My dear friend had just proofread the rough draft of my chapter and was trying to be as kind as possible. We met when our boys were in kindergarten together. Two little boys with autism. We didn't have a clue what the future would hold. It seems like a lifetime ago.

"And all the money you've spent on treatments with little to no help from insurance . . . I would write about that. Remember when they covered his probiotic, and then just quit?" she asked.

I remembered. Not just the cost of the treatments we paid for because they were not covered by insurance, but also the shock and judgment expressed when others heard we were using doctors and clinics that were not affiliated with the widely used mainstream hospitals nearby.

A million thoughts raced in my head, things I try to keep quiet about and not think of too often, like our mountain of credit card debt. I felt ashamed of it, even though I knew it was there for a good reason. I was healing my boy . . . and I really didn't care what it took to give him a chance at success.

"I remember when Tristen first started getting adjusted at the chiropractor, and you were like, 'You have to hear his speech!' After talking to him on the phone, I literally cried! I know, I'm a big baby," she laughed. The thing is, she wasn't. She is one of the strongest people I know, with the kindest heart. She loved Tristen from the first time she met him, and I felt the same way about her Caleb. "I'm not saying your rough draft isn't good." She paused. At that point, I knew our previous discussions about grammar and punctuation had been a stalling tactic. "But, I mean, your blog . . . is really good." *Aw, crap. I need to redo it.*

She laughed uncomfortably. I trusted her opinion. I needed her to be honest.

"Thank you," I replied. "I really needed to hear that! I am so nervous about writing this chapter! When I blog, I just write from my heart. I write what I'm feeling at that moment, and I don't really care who likes it and who doesn't. It's more of a therapeutic thing. But this . . . this is going to be right smack in the middle of dozens of amazing stories about autism written by brilliant, educated mother warriors. I don't know how I will measure up!" I went back to the computer to start from scratch.

I scanned the list of names. These ladies give their all, every day, to their family and their community. What have I gotten myself into? How do I fit in here? I thought about all the activism—the Facebook posts, the arguments, going toe-to-toe with the naysayers—but the sheer knowledge of these women seemed to far outweigh anything I'd been through. Needless to say, I was overwhelmed.

I was first drawn to the Thinking Moms' Revolution because I'd read about other moms who were living my life. I was interested not just because they were parents of children with autism, but also because they were "thinkers" and "doers." It seemed they knew all my inner thoughts and worst fears. And they were healing their kids, just like I was! They had read the same books and were determined, like I was, to get their kids healthy, despite the effort and cost. That was something I had never seen in any other autism parent in my community. People couldn't believe the lengths I would go to get treatment for my children; they thought I was crazy. But TMR showed me I wasn't.

So what makes me so special? Why would anyone want to hear my story, if it's just like the others? I am not the only one with more than one affected child, health issues of my own, or a limited income. I'm not even the only one with a husband with PTSD. What do I bring to the conversation?

Well, I can tell you what worked for my child. I can join the ranks in proclaiming that autism is treatable and that you can do it with limited means. I can share what has helped my son to make gains no one thought possible. I can prove that anyone with the correct information and determination can make a difference in the life of their child.

I'm a girl from a small farming community in the Midwest, where people trust their doctors. If something is not covered by insurance, they don't do it. It's cut and dried. My experience was different. I felt like I was screaming in the middle of a crowded room of doctors and barely anyone noticed. How could I help my child when no one would listen to me? Why was I always brushed off? Why didn't anyone care? Why didn't anyone see my child as a human being needing help instead of an "autistic"?

My son was injured at two days old by the hepatitis B vaccine. His perfect newborn cry turned into a jarring high-pitched scream. He couldn't latch on, causing me to bleed, and threw up most of what he ate. He would gulp down his food for a few short minutes, fall asleep, and wake up wailing. Sleep was only short catnaps, and he screeched every time he yawned. At his two-week checkup, he had a fever, so he was immediately admitted to the hospital and given strong antibiotics through an IV in his forehead. After three days of treatment, with all test results coming back negative, they sent us home without any answers or explanations.

Tristen spent the next two years sick with rashes, ear infections, sore throats, and fevers. We visited the doctor often, when the illnesses lasted for more than two weeks. After a quick exam and a strep culture, my concerns were quickly dismissed with a diagnosis of a viral infection. I was to go home and treat with Tylenol and try harder not to waste their time. I didn't understand how he could always be so sick without ever getting any additional testing or real attention from the doctors.

At Tristen's two-year check-up, I finally saw the doctor's concern I had been hoping for . . . except it was in the area of development. Up until this point, my little boy had progressed on schedule physically. The fact that he still had no words caused the doctor to study him a bit more and attempt to get his attention. He called Tristen's name and offered a treat and clapped. When Tristen did not respond, the doctor wrote a referral for a hearing test.

For the hearing test, he was to sit in a booth and look at lights and sounds. It was hard to keep him on my lap, but the lights helped, and he passed the test at the level that they were not concerned he was unable to hear. When the doctor read the results, we were immediately set up for an Early Intervention program called Birth to Three. It was at this point that I realized because of my focus on his illnesses, I had missed watching for his developmental milestones.

Just after the birth of my second child, I had the confirmation from the neurologist that my older son was on the autism spectrum. He did not have any language, make eye contact, or play with toys. He liked to line things up in a long row, kneel beside them, and put his head to the floor to look at them with one eye. Tristen was very determined, and when he had his mind set on something, it was nearly impossible to change it. I spent most of my energy redirecting and encouraging appropriate behavior.

At that time, I didn't even have a computer, let alone the Internet. In 2000, no one mentioned any support groups or books to read. A single piece of paper with a paragraph from the state Early Intervention program's speech pathologist, who was working with my nonverbal son, was the sole information I had on autism. So, I set out to really study my son to see how I could help him to learn and grow.

I had spent every minute with my child since birth. Much to the irritation of the maternity ward nurses, I wouldn't even let them take him from me for a bath or feeding. He was nursing so well (before the shot), and I didn't want to mess that up by having him bottle fed. I wanted to do it. They kept telling me I needed my rest, but I couldn't bear to be away from my newborn.

My husband worked nights and slept days, so I did it all. And I loved every minute of our time together. I wouldn't trade our bonding time for anything (of course, that doesn't mean it wasn't difficult to have a sick child). I believe that our time together helped me to understand him better. I knew every little detail about Tristen, what he wanted and when. I joked that he didn't need to talk because I knew what he wanted before he did. He never went to daycare and was very rarely watched by anyone else, and if so, it was only for about an hour. When he started Early Intervention, I soaked in everything they taught me and worked every day with him at every opportunity. I took the Hanen Program (More Than Words) when it was offered to me.

The Hanen Program taught me how to communicate with someone who was nonverbal by watching facial expressions, hand gestures, and body language. We discussed our challenges in the group and used videos to show examples of how to implement techniques. We had weekly assignments where we would practice a particular task with our child, like helping to bake cookies. I would do a "before" video and work all week on the task, and then do an "after" video. It was wonderful to see the progress after breaking down the task and creating steps to get ahead of the undesirable behavior. Using video recordings to critique our interactions gave me a new insight to understanding my son.

I didn't have Internet access in my home until my son was about three, and even then I didn't Google autism. I thought I knew what it was—if I had, I'm sure I would have made more connections back then. But what I didn't know was why my child was constantly sick. My poor boy missed so much school because of fevers and vomiting that I was frequently threatened with truancy. School was so important for him at this point because he needed the structure and the social interaction. Frustration set in as I questioned why I was trusting the doctors when it seemed they handed out Tylenol, Motrin, and Zyrtec like candy.

Living on an Army base was a new experience for us. One of the perks of being enlisted in the Army was having Tricare insurance with great coverage, as well as a base hospital close to home. It sounded perfect when my husband joined, but the reality looked a bit different—tired, overworked, and underpaid doctors with clinics always filled with patients because there was no co-pay. Patient care was lacking because the system was lacking, and we were slipping through the cracks. I needed to find someone to listen to me and run tests on my son, but I didn't know how.

My life was hectic with daily interventions for my son, all done as if I were a single parent because my husband was deployed more often than he was home. Tristen had a schedule board to list the events of the day like church, play dates, grocery shopping, playing at the park, and appointments. He went everywhere with me, and I treated each outing as a learning experience. From eating a meal sitting at the table using utensils to appropriate behavior at a birthday party, our plans were met with consistency and patience.

By 2007, I had had enough of doctors who didn't have answers, so I started to research illnesses. Not illnesses correlated with autism, but those that fit his symptoms in general. He had to have an underlying illness keeping him sick. I thought that if I found it, then I would know what to tell the doctors to test for. They would see that I was not a crazy, overprotective mother with nothing else to do but bother them.

I did hours and hours of research. Then I read about encephalopathy. It fit too perfectly. Before I was able to get back to the doctor to share my findings, something changed our lives forever. In October 2008, just by chance, my mother-in-law sent me a gift for my birthday, a book called *Changing the Course of Autism: A Scientific Approach for Parents and Physicians* by Bryan Jepson, MD. I hadn't heard of him before, but if a doctor had answers about autistic kids who were physically sick, I was all ears.

This book was about my son! This was exactly what I had been looking for! It had the answers to all my questions about his illness. The fevers, the vomiting, the constipation, the speech delays . . . I knew in that moment we *had* to find a Defeat Autism Now! doctor to treat Tristen for his chronic illness.

The nearest doctor was in Milwaukee, a good three-hour drive, but doable. I called ahead to find out the cost. We did not have any savings or any family to turn to for help. But it was time to make this happen. So first I had to get my husband to understand why we needed to add this extra expense and how I was going to pull it off. It went something like this:

Josh, the book your mom sent me? Well, it has all the answers to why Tristen is sick all the time—his fevers, his rashes—it even says the autistic symptoms get better as you treat the underlying conditions! I found a doctor who will do this stuff in Milwaukee. I was thinking that after we took away gluten and casein from Tristen's diet, he's been doing so much better. I said goodbye to him the other day when he left for the bus, like I've done every day since he was three, and for the first time, he turned back to look at me and said, "Bye, mom." I mean, I barely have to be at the school anymore, hardly ever get a phone call, and get all good notes from his teachers.

I waited for a reaction. He was a little interested. I kept going:

I saw in the paper I could be a substitute aide. They just call you when they need you. I think it would be perfect because if Tristen's sick or has a doctor appointment, I just wouldn't take a job that day. I think I could make about $80 a day because they don't prorate for the summer when you are a substitute. I should be able to save up enough money in no time to get him to see the doctor, and then it wouldn't add to our monthly bills. That way, we could afford it.

Clenching my jaw, I held my breath. "If you can save up the money to go, I don't see why not." Yes!

Money had always been tight. My husband tried to get work here and there for the first year of our marriage and soon realized he needed something more stable for our family. The Army had never been his ideal job, but he signed up and left for basic training on Tristen's first birthday. I was thrilled that he would be getting a steady paycheck, even if it was only $800 per month. He was only in the Army about six years before he was injured in Iraq. He came back with a crushed foot and was altered mentally and emotionally. PTSD (post-traumatic stress disorder) and TBI (traumatic brain injury) are similar to autism in the sense that they also seem to be a spectrum kind of disorder. They can be worse for some than others.

Even though he was honorably discharged because of a medical issue, we do not have the same privileges of a family with a retired member of the armed forces. He has an ID card so he can go onto any military base and use the VA clinic and hospital, and he can go to places like the commissary for grocery shopping at discounted prices. However, since I no longer have my ID card, his access doesn't help us—I do the family shopping as he is very busy with work. We also no longer have family insurance. My husband struggles just living in the world and being around people because it completely wears him out.

Over the years he tried numerous jobs from railroad to retail, which would go well for a while, and then he would fall apart due to mood swings and depression. When he finally decided to go to the VA, they prescribed him close to a dozen pharmaceuticals that caused stress to our family because of the side effects and the addictive nature of the drugs. The following years would prove very challenging as we fought to keep our heads above water.

Even though life was challenging, biomedical intervention was the only treatment for our son that made sense. Our son was physically ill, and learning that healing the underlying maladies would in turn help him to speak and learn gave us a hope and a plan for healing. No matter what it cost us, it would be worth it to have our special little boy healthy and happy. As parents, we felt we had no other choice but to do everything in our capacity to give him the chance at the best life.

During the years we spent struggling just to put food on the table, we were very blessed with some generous grants from NAA and the Angel Autism Network that helped us with biomedical interventions. Every little bit helped, and I will be forever grateful. For instance, we were able to start IV chelation, which pulled out large amounts of heavy metals from Tristen's body. At the time, Tristen had been at a first grade reading level for four years. Four months after this treatment, without any other interventions, he tested at a fourth grade level. We wanted to continue, but we had other expenses: his supplements cost $600 per month (and $300 more for his brother Tanner's supplements), so the grant money ran out just paying for their monthly regimen when we could not afford to.

We were also blessed to be part of a grant program for HBOT (hyperbaric oxygen therapy) in Madison. It was summer, and my husband was still out of work. We put the remaining expense on a Care Credit Card, used by only a few select number of doctors and clinics. We stayed at a friend's nearby home to reduce the cost of the treatments as much as possible. The HBOT helped, too. You could see it bringing old memories out of Tristen. It was as if you could watch his face and see how he was thinking and figuring out things that had never occurred to him before. He was talking so thoughtfully about things that happened when he was more severely affected by the autism and could not speak. With tears brimming his eyes and a soft crack in his voice, he told me that his kindergarten teacher had spanked him. "I was just a little boy. I just wanted to go home." It broke my heart. He had kept that inside for nine years, and although his communication skills had drastically improved, he had never shared that before. This made me even more determined to share his progress with the community. How many other children like my son who could not speak for themselves were being abused?

I also learned about a new program in our area called the Autism Whisperers Program offered at a Maximized Living chiropractic clinic. I was intrigued, and it was approved by our new insurance. The program was exactly like the biomed protocol, focusing on diet and supplements like we were used to, but added adjustments to the neck and spine—the missing piece to the puzzle. They also educated our family on toxins in food and the environment. The insurance later denied the coverage they had at first approved, but fortunately we were able to pay monthly.

After only a few adjustments, we noticed Tristen didn't "look" the same. He had always held his head back in a posturing sort of way so he was looking down his nose. Soon, he seemed more relaxed. His head rested comfortably on his neck, and he looked directly at us. After a week or so, someone commented that his head was finally looking proportional to his body. (Since he was a baby, he'd always had a large head.) His language and comprehension were becoming clear. He looked forward to his adjustments.

Progress came in slow spurts, but it continued upward. We couldn't be happier with our healthy boy, who had been free of any serious long-term illness for years and spending much more time in school. Because I worked the same school district my children attended, I saw what happened behind the scenes of the special education program and felt it didn't particularly fit Tristen's academic needs.

Being a special education teacher is challenging for many reasons, one of which being the spectrum of needs you are expected to meet. Often Tristen did not fit into a group and would either struggle with tasks that were too difficult or become complacent with tasks that were too simple. I needed to make a change, so I waited for the right opportunity.

During this time, we stayed gluten-, casein-, and soy-free, often using rice cakes in place of expensive GF breads or making our own sunbutter by blending sunflower seeds. In a pinch we would have homemade French fries and a plain hamburger patty for dinner. Sometimes our supplements were found in the clearance section or from Swanson Vitamins. The most important intervention we did, however, was using a schedule and remaining calm and consistent. Money cannot buy the results one gets from an attentive, patient parent.

In the summer of 2013, we moved to Texas—a big change. Dad was working again, giving me the opportunity to teach the boys at home instead of sending them to public school. This meant less family income than if we both worked, but we decided it was well worth the sacrifice. Tristen's academic level had not been close to his peers for quite a few years, making it difficult to place him in classes at his level. Often he was in classes that were too difficult, so he would rely on someone else to tell him what to write or he would copy notes from another student. I felt that teaching him at home would provide him with the opportunity to really learn at his level and at his own pace. Tristen has thrived in the homeschool environment, and we've explored so many of his interests and encouraged his talents. It has been a great blessing.

As my kids reach fourteen and sixteen years old, I am still teaching them so they can achieve their full potential. When I have money to invest, I go after every option that makes sense, and when I don't, I focus on good, clean, healthy food and necessary supplements. My main focus is teaching them what they need to know to succeed in life: honesty, integrity, dependability, and compassion, to name a few things. Hitting a low point doesn't mean it's over. There is always hope. I will do whatever it takes to heal my children and encourage them to be independent adults, regardless of the challenges and sacrifices. If it means I learn how to cut my own hair by watching YouTube tutorials, if it means my clothes come from the clearance rack at Wal-Mart, I never get a manicure or pedicure, I have to go to the food pantry, I drive a tiny Kia Rio because it's paid off, or even if I have to work nights and teach during the day, I will do it for my children. I never want to look back and regret what I didn't do for them. My time, my money, my sleep, my effort . . . my everything. They deserve it. Everything else is just "stuff."

Update

What a wild ride the past two years have been! Getting to know the Thinking Moms and spreading a message of hope and community has fulfilled my life in a unique way, and I am forever changed. Standing side by side with these strong, brilliant women, I can tell the world the truth about what happened to my children. Both my boys were injured by vaccines, and the doctors knew it, continued to vaccinate them, and refused to admit they were at risk. Since I wrote this chapter, my sisters became pregnant, and I realized in a very personal way why it is so important for us to get our government to hear us about what happened to our children. I shared with my family what I shared with the world because I don't want anyone to have to go through the heartache of seeing their child sick and in pain for years. It is heart-rending, and it doesn't need to happen. That's why I speak up.

Tristen is graduating from high school this spring. Taking the supplement EmPowerPlus, Brain Gain, and using the IonCleanse by AMD regularly dropped his ATEC (Autism Treatment Evaluation Checklist, a scale that indicates the severity of an individual's autism) score by over 40 points and turned my boy into a happy, healthy, confident young man who will be moving into his own apartment under our supervision. Although he still needs a schedule to remind him of daily tasks, Tristen told me he is ready for his life to begin.

"This *is* just the beginning, Tristen. The best is yet to come!"

14

Bling
Our Journey to Recovery

O N JANUARY 5, 2001, I GAVE BIRTH TO A BEAUTIFUL, HEALTHY baby boy named Gannon. It was a planned C-section delivery, and I was very calm and excited to meet my second son. When he rolled into my room in the hospital bassinet, I remember so clearly looking at him and being overwhelmed with the feeling that I needed to protect him. I called my friend who had three children and asked her if she had ever experienced this with any of her children's births. She told me that she had not, and I told her I was puzzled as to why I had this feeling with Gannon and not with my first-born son. I now know why—my son had a compromised immune system that I would not learn about for another four years.

Over the next nine months, Gannon developed normally, meeting all milestones ahead of or on schedule. He rolled over, sat up, crawled, and walked, all the while babbling, looking at us, and communicating with his sounds and his eyes.

Then, around his first birthday, we noticed that he was neither responding to our voices nor looking at us as much as he used to. Fast forward to his fifteen-month wellness visit with his pediatrician, when Gannon was given five vaccines. Over the next few months we noticed that he was losing more eye contact and no longer had solid stools. We also watched him become more agitated, and he stopped all progression with his speech.

He no longer turned his head when we called his name, and he seemed very socially disconnected. I remember taking him to our "mom and tot" class and noticing that he was the only child who could not sit still at circle time. He also did not play with any of the other children in his class; instead, he ran off. I get exhausted thinking about having to run after him and bring him back to the circle only to find him running away again after I sat down.

I asked my pediatrician about this behavior, as well as his lack of speech and loose, very smelly stools. He responded that Gannon's loose stools were the result of him eating a lot of fruit and that his lack of speech was due to the fact that he was a boy and boys began talking later than girls. *What?* I was uneducated at the time, so I had no idea how to question him more effectively. We had *no clue* as to what was happening to our son.

At the age of three, we had him evaluated by our local school. After his testing was completed, we were told that he was "speech- and language-impaired" and we needed to enroll him in an early education classroom. Attending the school required our boy to be taken away on a bus every morning—according to the school, the bus would help eliminate his anxiety and reduce his inattentive run- ning, which was occurring on a daily basis. I was completely shocked when I heard this stipulation. He was only three! I was frightened and sad.

After he began attending his ECDD (Early Childhood Developmental Delay) classroom, his behaviors actually got worse! He was biting and pushing little girls; he was also becoming even more anxious. Phone calls alerting me to Gannon's distressing behaviors were becoming a daily occurrence. I was afraid to answer the phone because I did not want hear any more bad news. Then it happened: the phone call from his teacher telling me she suspected Gannon had autism and we needed to get him evaluated. *What?* Part of me died at that moment. During this same time, my older son was experiencing extreme separation anxiety in kindergarten, and I had also given birth to our third child, a little girl who refused to take a bottle and was attached to me for a good part of the day. I had no help during the night for feedings because my husband couldn't feed her. My world was crashing. I remember pulling over into a church parking lot and saying out loud, "God, I know you won't give me more than I can handle . . . *Well, I can't handle any more . . . I am going to die!*"

I picked myself up, recharged and ready to fight. Yes, the Lord had answered my prayers and given me more strength! I dove into research, looking for testimonies and ideas that could help my family. I noticed that diet kept coming up on many of the Internet sites that I visited. Something that really stood out to me was gluten intolerance, because my sister-in-law had just been diagnosed with it and said she never knew how sick she felt until she removed the gluten and saw the improvement—she had grown up feeling ill and had come to view it as "normal." I thought, *what if my poor little boy is in pain and he doesn't know how sick he is or can't communicate it to me?*

All right, let's clean out the pantry! I removed all gluten, sugar, and artificially flavored/colored products from our pantry and called his teacher to let her know that Gannon would be following a strict diet. He was not allowed any food other that what I sent for him. There was a moment of silence on the phone after I gave my instructions, and then I heard, "Mrs. Scheer, I just need to tell you that there is no scientific proof that a special diet will help Gannon." I told her that I didn't need scientific proof, I needed proof from families that had experienced improvements through diet. Well, this turned out to be one of our most important protocols. Within three months, our baby spoke his first complete sentence. That sentence was "I love you too, mommy!" I felt so much *joy*. We knew that we were on the right track, and that same teacher now told us that she has become a believer in the gluten-free diet after witnessing Gannon's speech explode and his ability to potty train finally take off.

Over the next two years, working with our DAN! (Defeat Autism Now!) doctor, we implemented protocols for yeast, bacteria, and viruses that included many natural supplements as well as pharmaceutical medications. He was soon speaking more; however, he was still a runner and full of pain and anxiety. He would scream if he heard singing and was continuing to bite and push other children down. He was unable to walk into a movie theater due to severe sensory issues, and he was also a very picky eater. We couldn't go anywhere in public with him for fear that we would lose him. He was fast on his feet and could vanish in only a moment's time. He knew no fear and would go away with anyone. We became prisoners in our own home.

I needed help, so I found an autism support group meeting. Off I went. I walked into a room with about twenty moms who had children with autism. Throughout the evening, I saw photos of children at Disney World and heard about adventures at Chuck E. Cheese. I left the meeting, got in my car, and *cried my eyes out*. Disney and Chuck E. Cheese . . . how? We couldn't even think of going to any of these places because our son might hurt another child, get lost, or go with a stranger and never some back. I felt so alone—I didn't even fit in at an autism support meeting.

Again, I prayed for help—and help did arrive. I later found another group with families more like ours, and I finally felt like I was not the only person alive going through this.

Time went on. Age five and a half brought our worst day ever. (Don't worry . . . this story has a happy ending. I just need to let you know about the bad so that you can truly understand how far we've come. Later we will celebrate the good!)

It was a summer day, and I was upstairs doing laundry. My phone rang, and a lady on the other end said, "I have your son." *What?* I lost my breath for a moment and then started running through the house to find Gannon. My last stop was the back door, and there I found two boxes stacked up. Gannon had put them there to climb on and release the dead bolt. He was *gone*! The lady then told me that she was at the entrance to our subdivision with Gannon. I jumped on my bicycle and raced to the front of our sub, which is three blocks from our home. When I approached, I saw two police cars, four police officers, and my son in his underwear, no shoes, no clothing. I ran up to Gannon and picked him up. My mind was racing. Was the police officer going to question my parenting, was he going to take Gannon from me, what was going to happen? I must have had a horrified look on my face, because when I made eye contact with one of the officers, he nodded that it was okay for me to leave with my son.

I took Gannon home and put him on the couch to talk to him. He was like an empty shell, like someone had stolen his soul. He had no fear, no remorse, and no idea what had just happened. I remember saying, "Gannon, where are you?" He mumbled the words, "I don't know." I left the room and sobbed. I was numb with worry of what the future would hold for him. I knew we had to do more for this child!

It was now time for kindergarten, but we had no idea where to enroll our son. We searched and searched, and finally decided to try him in a Christian school. Well, it did not go well at all! He was screaming, wandering, and biting. One day at recess, he took off and was found biting the metal fence at the edge of the school property. The teacher was not equipped to handle Gannon, and it was very obvious that we needed to move him. Next stop was a kindergarten classroom with a one-on-one aid. This did not work either. He was throwing chairs, eating dirt, and urinating on the playground! The stress level in my body was reaching an all-time high, and I needed to find a solution.

I spoke with the consultant for school district's program for autistically impaired children. They told me about an incredible teacher in another school who ran an emotionally impaired (EI) classroom. *Really?* I did not want my son in a classroom with children who are going to teach him *more* bad behaviors! She assured me, however, that this would be a great fit for Gannon—this particular class had two children with autism as well as nine other children with only mild behavioral problems. She assured me that the teacher had a handle on things. Feeling frightened and insecure about this recommendation, I called the director of special education at our school district and left an urgent message regarding this new classroom. I left three messages total and then decided to call the superintendent, because I knew there was only one spot left in this classroom, and I needed to get it for my son. Sometimes you need to go to the top to get things done, and when it's your child, you can't hold back.

I set up a meeting with the head teacher in the EI classroom. Gannon and I went to check it out. I told her ahead of time that Gannon had become obsessed with the color blue and elephants and I needed a teacher that was strong enough to not to give in to his obsessions. He had to have the blue ball, the blue scooter, the blue pencil, and anything else that was blue. He also had to have the elephant if his class was doing anything with animals. And if he didn't get the color or animal he wanted, he would scream. Everyone at the other two schools was catering to his outbursts to keep as much peace as possible, which was not teaching him anything. He needed a teacher who would teach him that he could not always get what he wanted.

She immediately challenged him by giving him a carpet square with a giraffe on it, knowing that he would explode because it was not the elephant. She handled him beautifully, so I knew this was the place for our Gannon. Her calm, yet firm approach was just what he needed. Finally, after three schools in three months, we had found our home! Gannon would be learning to cope with situations that did not go his way, and how to remain calm and walk away from situations that were making him upset.

Meanwhile, I continued my own research, looking for new approaches. I went to a DAN! conference and heard a parent panel speak about chelation. (Chelation is the process of removing heavy metals from the body and can be done orally, transdermally, or intravenously.) There was one mom who stood out to me after she showed the before and after video of her son. Her son reminded me of Gannon. Seeing the results, I knew that this was a therapy that we were now ready to try. During the next two years, we were fortunate to see many improvements. Gannon's world was opening up to other interests, and his anxiety level was dropping. He could now sit with the family while we sang "Happy Birthday" and not run screaming out of the room.

We then added hyperbaric oxygen therapy (HBOT), along with more new supplements, and saw even more improvements. We went to the movie theater for the first time ever without Gannon running out with his hands over his ears. In fact, when we walked into the theater, Gannon went down to the front of the screen, spread his hands out, and said, "This is great!" He was also able to ride his bike without training wheels, which he would never even consider trying just four months prior. He also made his way into the swimming pool for the first time ever. His fear of water had subsided. He used to run around the outside edge of the pool while all the other children played, but now he was going in with a swim toy and kicking his legs all around the pool. He was making gains every day!

Things were moving along greatly. He was in third grade now, and he was spending about twenty minutes each day in a general education classroom. He gradually increased his time in general ed to an hour each day, and then to two hours. We were very happy with his success; however, he still needed to become more independent and more socially aware and mature. We were switching things up with his protocols, but somewhere along the way, we became stuck. We did not have any notable improvements over the next three years.

We later began working with an internal medical specialist to go after pathogens and parasites. About a month into his treatment, we were amazed that our son began to move forward again. His social skills increased tenfold! He was complimenting me, asking to help with chores, and becoming more responsible at school. *Wow!* With this protocol, we attended a social gathering, and Gannon came back to the table and said, "Mom, I just did a good deed."

"Really, what did you do?"

"I was at the drink table and someone came up to the table, so I poured their juice for them."

Next we went to a roller-skating party with his school, and Gannon, who could barely stand up on skates, announced to us that he was going to be in the race! *Holy cow.* I was freaked out and happy at the same time. I did not want to discourage him; however, I did not want him to get run over, either. The race began, and we cheered wildly from the sidelines, "Go Gannon, go!" Of course he came in last place, so I made my way over to the other end of the rink to make sure he wasn't going to have a meltdown because he didn't win. The way Gannon handled defeat was one of our biggest struggles— he simply could not handle losing. Well, not only did he maintain his composure, he skated up to me and said, "It's okay that I didn't win, Mom. I had fun." I wanted to call *Good Morning America* right then and tell them that I had just witnesses a miracle.

We later began working with an infectious disease specialist who added stronger anti-parasitic medications to his schedule, and again, huge gains abounded. He had now graduated from his self-contained EI classroom and was with his typical peers all day long. We were thrilled! We continued his other treatments as well. We did forty dives in a hard-sided HBOT chamber and saw more incredible gains. He was now asking for different foods and was not having attacks of anxiety. His busy days of school, math tutoring, and HBOT were being handled with ease and happiness. He became so responsible with his homework and did not get upset when we asked him to do it. In fact, he would go to his room and do it independently. Again, *wow*! He became the star of his school talent show with his choreographed rendition of "Banana Phone" and was moved onto a competitive baseball team at the Miracle League of Michigan. His social skills in school were still lacking, but he was well loved by his peers. His personality was shining through. Telling jokes became his hobby, and at his fifth grade graduation he was awarded "Funniest Student" in the class elections.

This brings us to September 2013. Middle school! To say we were nervous would be a huge understatement. I was a complete wreck. Middle school is scary enough for any child, let alone one who had been through so much. Luckily, he had shadowed a student during the prior school year's orientation and really liked what was to be his new school. He was excited to get out of his elementary school.

I'll never forget my thoughts on the first day. I felt like I was releasing him to the wolves. I was so afraid! We went to orientation, and then we went back in a couple of days before school began. We practiced his locker combination and his classroom route several times. Finally, he said he was ready. I realized that Gannon's locker was on the opposite end of the sixth grade hall and that he would probably have a hard time getting to his classes on time. I did not say anything to his teachers, as I wanted to try my hardest not to be a "helicopter parent." On the third day of school, Gannon came home and told us that he had been given a new locker, so we needed to go in early the next day to learn his new combination. Gannon and I went to school early the next day.

As we were approaching the lockers, I glanced down the hall to see locker number 54. A handicapped locker with a bright blue sign on it! It took all my strength not to burst into tears! I immediately began to peel the sticker off and I remained very calm for

Gannon. The look on his face nearly broke my heart. After years of just wanting to fit in with everyone else, he had this locker that said that he's handicapped. They may as well have had a big blinking light on it, too!

A teacher walked by and told me that I was not allowed to remove the sticker because they had to have a certain number of lockers in the school for handicapped children. "Well, we don't need it, so it's coming off," I said. I then looked at Gannon, and I'll never forget the words that came from his mouth. As he shrugged his shoulders and took a breath, he said, "It's okay, Mom, it's just a sticker. I know I'm not handicapped." I said, "You're right Gannon, it's no big deal." My beautiful son had handled this situation better that I did. Of course, I kept it all inside, so as not to upset him. However, this time he was perfectly fit to handle a tough situation all by himself.

I went to the parking lot and sobbed. I was sad and happy at the same time, and so proud of my son! I called the principal and apologized for taking off the sticker. He told me not to worry about it. He felt very bad about what had happened, explaining that they just gave him a number from a list, not knowing that it was a handicapped locker. He offered Gannon another locker, but Gannon decided to keep the one he was given. "It's bigger than the others and easier to get my stuff in and out of," he said. "I think I'll keep it." I later noticed that all the handicapped stickers were removed from the larger lockers in the school.

I will end this chapter with the words that Gannon spoke when he was near recovery. We were walking along the monuments in Washington, DC, when he walked up to me, put his arm around me, and shared these words with me. These are his exact words:

Thank you for being the best mom in the world
You love me and you heal me
What would I ever do without you
I want to go back in time to the good old days when I was little

I am remembering those times
When I was an infant and you held me all the time
Oh, Mom, please don't ever leave this world
I love you so much.

These are the words of a child who has beaten the odds and won his nine-year battle with autism. He has "woken up," and he has taught our family more in the past ten years than we could have learned in a whole lifetime.

I will be forever grateful for the support, encouragement, and tireless help of my loving husband, kids, and Gannon's grandparents. I give all the glory to God for our strength and our son's recovery.

Praise to you, Lord Jesus Christ!

Update

First, let me say how enthusiastic I am for the opportunity to share our "what happened next" story in the updated edition of our book! And thank you for reading and seeking out information for yourself and your child.

The most exciting information is that Gannon experienced absolutely NO regression while continuing on through puberty. This is important to note, because heartbreakingly, many children on the autism spectrum experience regression during these years. I will be honest and say that I sometimes feel guilty about sharing this information in my close-knit autism circles, because I know many moms who are going through intensely difficult times with their teenage children. We are among the lucky ones. We have no explanation of why Gannon is handling puberty so well. We just continue to be grateful and share the message that recovery is possible! We pray for him every day, and we also visualize his wellness and accomplishments.

We continue his clean, gluten-free diet (with very little dairy), and we give him vitamin and mineral supplements to keep him strong. We also see a natural healer. We are incredibly blessed to have an amazing pediatrician who sees Gannon annually and runs tests to make sure that his body is running as it should. The one fantastic tool we've added is the IonCleanse footbath by AMD. This is a fantastic way (in my opinion) to gently detox him, as well as the entire family, removing all the nastiness we are exposed to in our everyday environments. Gannon enjoys his foot baths (as do I), and is now learning how to set them up and do them himself.

As far as the physical improvements go, we have continued to see weight gain, increased muscle tone, and an increased appetite. Gannon is now a 5'10" eighth grader, with the strength to row himself across the lake in his own kayak. He also bowls three games a week on his youth bowling league.

Now let's get on to the really cool things!

Four months after our first book was published, Gannon began seventh grade with a bang. He came home and told us that he had decided to run for student council representative and, at the last minute, went down to the office to give his "Vote for Me" speech over the loud speaker. At the end of the day, he was notified that he had won one of the positions and would be a student council representative for his seventh grade class of over 350 students.

In March of that school year, Gannon joined the forensics team to compete in public speaking and chose the category of storytelling. As I sat in the back of the very quiet judging room, I kept thinking to myself, *these judges have NO IDEA of the miracle they are witnessing.* He blew us away with his confidence and proved his early doctors wrong once again—the boy who "may never speak a sentence" was competing in the field of *public speaking!*

Now we move on to the most amazing year of Gannon's life so far. He was a big eighth grader, and his goal was to try out for a role in the school play, *The Lion King Jr.* Not just any role—one of the *lead* roles! We were all excited and helped him practice his song and run his lines until the big audition day. Our daughter had also decided to try out for many roles, including the role that Gannon really wanted. We shared with them the importance of supporting each other and coached them on how to accept the director's choice as a professional decision, not taking anything personally. I will be honest and tell you that I was a complete mess as I sat outside in the hallway listening in on their auditions. This was the largest audition his school had ever seen, with nearly 100 students trying out. *Oh, Lord!* I prayed constantly. I asked everyone I knew to pray. And then we waited . . .

Thank goodness we did not know the exact date they would be posting the cast list, because if we had, I would have never been able to concentrate on anything that day. A few days later, I left town to participate in the Autism Education Summit in Dallas, Texas. On the second day of the conference, I received a text from my husband that read, "CALL GANNON NOW!"

I was sitting at the Autism Hope Alliance booth when I received the message. I called back, and he picked up the phone and said, "Hi Mom, I got Timon!" Needless to say, I *lost it*, and began to cry. I heard him say, "Mom, are you okay?"

"Yes, Gannon, I am fine. I am just so excited and happy for you!"

He then told me his sister got the role of Shenzi the Hyena, and I began to sob. Of course, I wished I had been there with my family to celebrate in person; however, I felt incredibly blessed to be in the presence of some of my dearest friends and warrior moms at that moment. My dear friend Kristin and Team TMR sisters Lone Star and Juicy Fruit also happened to be right near me. They hugged me and joined in the celebration—they knew our story and realized what a miracle this was. I had to leave the booth and collect myself. I went and shared the news with Shawty, another Team TMR sister, and a few other warrior mom friends who were also at the conference. I knew right then that there was a reason I found out while I was at the conference: to share this message of hope with the many moms and dads who would visit our booth over the next two days.

The Icing on the Cake

Of course, my entire family was so excited for the play, and we all got involved. I joined the makeup, hair, and costume committees. My husband and father joined the set design committee, and everyone offered to help in any way they could.

I will never forget the first committee meeting I attended. We were in a room that shared a wall with the stage, and I could hear one of Gannon's scenes. I completely zoned out of the conversation with my group and listened to his voice on the other side of the wall. Then I looked at the other moms and said to myself, *they have no idea there is a miracle happening on the other side of this wall.* I felt paralyzed and completely separated, as if I were standing alone, away from anyone who knew anything about us. None of these women knew about Gannon's struggles or our ten years of therapies, protocols, and endless doctor appointments. They had no idea.

Over the next two months, we rehearsed and rehearsed. I was concerned about the hours Gannon was spending rehearsing, and I was always bringing him healthy snacks and lots of water to keep his body going. He sailed through the rehearsals and was makings new friends! During rehearsals, I would sneak out to take a look at the kids, and I was excited to see Gannon hanging with a table of guys playing games and having fun with each other. My heart was happy.

When show week began, my anxiety increased as the directors were offering much more criticism to tighten the show up. I was worried about how Gannon would handle the feedback. I was always trying to make sure he never saw any of my stress, because I did not want him to pick up on anything I was feeling. I was constantly telling myself to let him go and experience this without me towering over him. That was one of the toughest things I've ever had to do. I was there, but I was letting him own it, allowing him to soar.

Opening night came. His practitioner suggested upping his vital nutrients to help with his energy; she also told me to keep myself calm—yeah, right! I was backstage helping everyone with makeup and costumes, and then running through the back hallway to get glimpses of the show from the back of the auditorium. Gannon and his sister were rocking it! It was a dream come true for both of them, and they were experiencing it together! I was reminded of the time that Gannon was so ill he didn't even know his sister existed. And now they were sharing a true "brother-sister" bond like never before.

Over the next few days, I received text messages, phone calls, emails, and Facebook messages from friends, family, and teachers who had seen the show. Everyone was amazed by his timing, energy, clarity, and his connection with the audience. One Facebook message read, "I heard Gannon was the star of the show last night!" *Wowza!* And the best was yet to come . . .

Two days after the show opened, I received a friend request from the head of the theater department of one of the high schools in our area. This school is known for their incredible theatrical performances year after year in our community. I accepted his request and soon received this message: "I just wanted to say hi and let you know how proud I was of your son's performance. Of course, I must ask you to consider sending your boy to Western, so he can be a part of our choirs and musical theater program."

I am crying again now as I write this. I can't even put into words all the emotion that flooded my body. I ran to my husband, who is a professional performer, and showed him. He had tears in his eyes as he said, "Our boy is being recruited!"

Yes, all those years of therapies, diets, protocols, doctor visits, pain, and desperation had brought us to this moment in time: the day our boy defied the odds and accomplished far beyond what the experts told us he would accomplish!

So, at the beginning of our journey, Gannon could not speak a sentence, and now he is competing in public speaking, starring in his middle school musical, and being recruited for theater.

I'll say it again: "Praise to you, Lord Jesus Christ!"

Always remember, hope is real and recovery *is* possible!

Love, hugs, and blessings.

15

Cougar
Recovery Is Possible

RECOVERY IS POSSIBLE! WE ARE DESIGNED TO HEAL, AND WILL heal if given the opportunity. Don't let anyone tell you otherwise. The underlying causes of disease, including the symptoms known as autism, are a result of toxicity, an acidic body, and lack of oxygen to the cells. All of these things can be addressed and reversed, leaving "autism" behind. My son is living proof that there is hope.

My son's journey into and out of autism began over ten years ago, when my husband and I found out I was pregnant. We were thrilled! The nursery was perfect. The baby shower was perfect. I felt great throughout the nine months of pregnancy. Our baby boy was developing normally. At the time, I considered us healthy eaters. We were eating a vegetarian diet with some fish. (Fish is known to be a source of mercury, and we don't eat it now, nor did I eat any seafood with my next three pregnancies. Other than the fish I ate when pregnant, I had no other source of mercury. I did not even have metal fillings in my mouth, and did not get a RhoGAM shot, which does contain injected mercury.) Overall, the pregnancy was easy and enjoyable.

My son was born in September 2003 via an uneventful, routine C-section. He had normal APGAR scores, good hearing, and normal reflexes. He was a healthy, beautiful, bright blue-eyed, strawberry blond boy. On the day of his birth, Christopher was given an injection of synthetic vitamin K and a HepB vaccination. We had not researched either of these injections, but were just following the normal procedures with a hospital birth. After those injections, our son became jaundiced. We were clueless as to the reason for the jaundice, and we just accepted the explanation from the hospital's pediatrician that his liver needed to develop more. I now know that jaundice is a clear indicator that the liver is overtaxed.

Who decided that all babies need a large injection of synthetic vitamin K? Why are we injecting every child with HepB—a disease that affects less than 1 percent of our population? The two at-risk groups for contracting hepatitis B are adult, promiscuous homosexual males and IV drug users who share needles. A day-old baby fits neither of these two categories. Why was my son injected with two things that we were not fully informed about by those administering the injections?

Our first night home with Christopher was bittersweet. Sweet because we had this wonderful little person who was now a part of our family; bitter because he had feeding issues. The frenulum under his tongue was connected all the way to the tip. None of the lactation consultants had noticed this because he latched well. He would latch, but was unable to extract milk. The first night at home he screamed from hunger almost the entire night while we "finger-fed" him formula. I was in pain, and the finger feeding was ridiculous! The next day, he went from a breastfed baby to a formula-fed baby. We were "healthy" eaters, and I had just finished a super baby food book that listed healthy ways to feed a baby. This book promoted soy, and since we were already dairy-free in our diet, Christopher began soy formula.

I was not informed that soy formula is basically poison. It's especially bad for boys because of its estrogen-mimicking properties. Ninety-eight percent of soy is genetically modified, so when the soy fields are sprayed with poisonous pesticides, it's the only thing that remains. This formula made my son chronically constipated. We discussed the problems with his pediatrician, who told us to add corn syrup to every bottle. I'll never forget this appointment. We waited for a half hour to see her for less than eight minutes of her time. She commented, "How cute," noticed his tongue tie (she said that we just needed "to watch it"), and recommended corn syrup for the constipation. She ended with, "The nurse will be in with his vaccines." Christopher was only weeks old and was eating poisonous soy formula with added corn syrup from a Dr. Brown's BPA-filled plastic bottle that I had dipped in boiling tap water to sterilize. All of this was the backdrop for his vaccine injury.

I could write an entire book on vaccines because of the last eight years of research I've done and my personal experience with a vaccine-injured child. I could tell you how and why they do not provide immunity, the history of them all the way back to Edward Jenner, the stories of thousands of other parents whose children were also harmed (some of those babies died after just one vaccine). For now, I'll just give you my favorite vaccine quote as food for thought. It comes from Rebecca Corley, MD, VIDS (vaccine-induced diseases) expert:

> What the promoters of vaccination fail to realize is that the respiratory tract of all mammals contain secretory IgA within the respiratory tract mucosa. By passing this mucosa aspect of the immune system directly injecting organism leads to a corruption of the immune system. As a result, pathogenic viruses or bacteria cannot be eliminated by the immune system and remain in the body where they further grow and/

or mutate as the individual is exposed to ever more antigens and toxins in the environment. This is especially true
with viruses grouped under the term "stealth adapted." The
immune system is corrupted when you understand the two
poles of the immune system (the cellular and the humoral
mechanism) have reciprocal relationship. Thus when one is
stimulated the other is inhibited. Since vaccines activate the
B cells to secrete antibody, the T-Cells are subsequently sup-
pressed. This suppression of the cell mediated response is a
key factor in the development of cancer and life threatening
infections . . .

How did vaccination affect Christopher? His gut was a mess
from all the soy and corn syrup. That was the underlying factor for
why he couldn't detox all the known neurotoxins in the vaccines he
received. He had high-pitched screaming with both hands up by his
ears immediately after each vaccine. This was a sign of neurological
damage. The pediatrician was completely clueless about this response
and never even considered this to be a sign of a vaccine reaction. We
ended up leaving the pediatrician's practice because a light bulb had
finally gone off. We questioned why we were giving Christopher all
that corn syrup—something we wouldn't eat ourselves.

We were slowly waking up. We went to a new pediatrician who
did not agree with the corn syrup method. This pediatrician appeared
to be more informed. We were still vaccinating on schedule, however,
and Christopher still had the high-pitched screaming reaction each
time. Somewhere before the nine-month well-baby visit, someone at
work had planted a seed in my husband's mind that maybe all these
vaccines weren't so great. We asked the new pediatrician about it,
and he assured us that he had read everything and that our worries
were unfounded. He talked us into keeping on schedule, a decision
we will forever regret. Christopher screamed after that nine-month
set of vaccines for forty minutes until he passed out. The next day, he

projectile-vomited his soy formula across the living room. He wasn't the same after that well visit.

Soon, Christopher started having OCD-type behaviors where he would repeat the same motion over and over. He lost eye contact. He started staring into space for hours while twisting his wrists and ankles. Some family members would comment that he was "so well-behaved," but he was in a fog. He stopped responding to his name. He did not develop language typically. He had no comprehension of what was said to him. He did not interact socially with other children, and he had daily meltdowns over nothing. He always had to hold something and would freak out if it was dropped, even if the object was given back to him. His stool was never normal. He went from constipation to liquid orange stool that smelled like alcohol. In many ways, this was not the same happy, attentive, alert baby we once had.

All parents have special memories of their children's major life events, like the first birthday and the first day of preschool. This is what I remember from Christopher's early years: At his first birthday, he was in a fog. He sat in his high chair with the little cake made just for him and stared into space. One of his grandmothers kept calling his name and put his hand in the cake. We wanted him to dig into the cake on his own like one-year-olds are supposed to do. That never happened, nor did it happen at his second birthday. He was unaware of the gifts right in front of him and didn't tear them open at his first birthday, first Christmas, or his second birthday.

I remember taking him to the park when he was twenty-six months old with his cousins, their friends, and my sister-in-law. All the other kids were interacting, having fun. Christopher was walking on the sidewalk that went around the perimeter of the park, staring at the ground directly in front of him, not responding to his name. I spent the entire day following behind him so that he didn't wander off. When we left, I had to pick him up and carry him to the car while he kicked and screamed. He screamed from the moment I lifted him until he finally passed out in the car seat, a half hour later.

For the most part, Christopher was in a fog, often completely unaware of his surroundings. He would be happy in his little fog, and then some random thing would happen that sent him into meltdown mode. Meltdown mode is not your typical kid tantrum. These meltdowns are over absurd things, and they can last up to an hour or even longer. Our family made a trip to Target once and Christopher wasn't holding anything in his hands, so he fixated on a blue bottle of carpet spray. We were not there to purchase carpet spray, so we left without it. My husband ended up carrying Christopher out to the car under his arm while our son screamed and kicked. Our little guy just didn't understand what was going on. We stopped at a drug store on the way home, bought a blue bottle of carpet cleaner, and the meltdown stopped. Another day, my husband was taking out the trash, and Christopher didn't understand what was happening. So he had a forty-five-minute meltdown. There was no amount of consoling that would stop this type of behavior. This was not normal.

Another memory etched in my mind is that of Christopher having a seizure. A family member wearing some kind of tanning cream on her skin hugged him, and he immediately broke out in a red, swollen rash. The pediatrician was called and told us to give our son Benadryl, which caused a seizure. Christopher was unable to focus on us and ended up with his eyes rolling back in his head. Although he has had that type of seizure only once, he has also had several absence seizures. During an absence seizure, the person is stuck. It's like the body freezes for a minute or two before the person snaps out of it.

Despite these difficulties, there were good memories even during the bad times. For instance, Christopher had always been a tender-hearted, loving boy!

At twenty-one months old, Christopher was still having feeding issues, partly because he had an aversion to the textures of certain foods. The tongue tie was still a problem as well. He couldn't fully move his tongue. An ENT put him to sleep to clip his tongue. "The tongue tie was so thick," the ENT told me, "that's why you couldn't breast-feed." Christopher was not yet three at the time of this surgery, so our state Early Steps Program sent an occupational therapist to our home to work with him on eating. At this point, we knew something wasn't "right" with Christopher, but because he was our first child, we weren't sure exactly what. The OT eventually became a friend and told us that on the first day that she met Christopher, she knew he had autism.

At twenty-eight months, per the OT's recommendation, we had Christopher evaluated by a person from the state. I will never forget that day. The testing was done at our home. My son had such poor motor skills that he couldn't even jump. It never occurred to him to climb the steps to his bunk bed, nor to slide down the other side. He had no comprehension of what this state social worker was saying to him. She asked, "Christopher, can you hand me the blue ball?" The ball was right beside him on the floor, and he just stared blankly at her. She repeated the question three or four times, finally handing him the ball, to which he robotically said, "blue ball."

His scores were around a nine-month-old level almost across the board, and he was declared developmentally delayed. It was at nine months that he had had that horrific vaccine reaction.

When a child is declared "delayed," "autistic," or anything related, the parent is a crying mess, like I was, but the people doing the evaluating are not there for comfort. With so many children having a learning and/or developmental delay, the evaluators must become numb to it all. The day Christopher was declared delayed, I got a "You'll be okay" as the person was walking out.

When most of the crying was over, it was time to devise a plan of action. The state had officially declared him delayed, so he was now eligible for more services from our state's Early Intervention program, starting at age three. Without getting to the root cause of the neurological damage, all the help was not enough. The speech therapy and Special Ed instruction provided through any state are very limited. Christopher got one half-hour speech therapy session with a group at a local school. In addition, a Special Ed teacher came to work with him at our home for a half hour, three days a week, which was quickly reduced to two days a week because of limited instructors. This was from 2006 to 2008. One can only imagine how limited state-sponsored interventions are today, given that one in six children is now diagnosed with a learning, behavioral, or developmental delay.

Rather than pay out of pocket for extra therapy, we chose to pay out of pocket for biomedical intervention. We decided, after extensive research and talking with others that were very knowledgeable about what we were facing, our first stop would be a local DAN! doctor. We waited six months to get an appointment. We spent approximately three thousand dollars on that visit. This included a fee for the appointment, tests that were ordered, a blood analysis on a microscope, a truckload of supplements, and our first batch of compounded B12 injections. This was just the beginning both of Christopher's journey to recovery and the cost of this journey. We have currently spent the equivalent of a college education on him, and he's worth every penny.

We were also fortunate to have very supportive family members, to whom we are forever grateful! On the day of our initial appointment, my husband's aunt slipped us one thousand dollars. My in-laws have paid for countless supplements, and my parents have purchased many other things we needed, all without question. We spent more per month on food and supplements than on our mortgage. We are truly fortunate that we were able to afford the biomedical treatments that Christopher needed to recover.

The test results were back after a few weeks, and here is what we saw: mercury, aluminum (both vaccine ingredients), and lead levels were all off the charts; there was also a horrible bacterial infection in his gut, and yeast everywhere. His blood analysis under the microscope showed his red blood cells to be deflated in the middle, more kidney shaped than round, and clumped together. Behind the clumped blood cells were small white strings, which the doctor said was undigested food. On the undigested food was yeast that looked like cotton candy. The doctor commented that most of the autistic kids she sees have this condition.

Based on the results, we did the following biomedical interventions: daily MB12 injections from a compounding pharmacy for two years, then B12 nasal spray after that, 105 CaEDTA chelation IVs, removal of all wheat, dairy, and soy from our diets, HBOT, infrared sauna, and a spreadsheet of daily supplements. The spreadsheet was empowering, and every time we checked off the supplement that was given to our son, we knew that he would recover. For the chelation IVs, my husband took off work every Thursday morning and we drove to the doctor's office as a family. The DAN! doctor and her staff became close friends and would ask us to speak to parents who were there for the first time.

I cried a lot during that season. For the most part, the autistic kids in our country are hidden. At school, the majority are in their own classrooms. Many of the parents can't go to a restaurant or shopping with them. It was very sobering to see what these DAN! doctors do. I remember meeting a mom with beautiful two-and-a-half-year-old twin girls. One was talking and playing with my daughter, while the other twin stared blankly into space. The mom told me that their pediatrician had accidentally vaccinated one girl twice with MMR, while the other got no MMR. I've heard this same account of vaccine reaction causing autism a thousand times. But every week hearing these accounts still made me cry.

Christopher's progress on his biomedical protocol was slow and steady. When we removed the soy, wheat, and dairy, his fog lifted. He started looking at us directly rather than out of the corner of his eye. As we removed the metals from his body, he started to engage us more; he also started losing his sensory issues. He would now eat solid food, rather than just applesauce, yogurt, and other soft foods. He stopped labeling things, "cup, book, mommy," and started echolalia. (Echolalia is when the child knows they should respond to what was said or asked of them but doesn't know what to say, so they repeat the last thing said to them; it can also be just repetition of familiar words or phrases.)

At the time, Christopher was enrolled in a three-days-a-week preschool program. When I picked him up in the afternoon, I would ask, "What did you do today?" to which he would respond in a robotic voice, "Did you paint a green frog?" I would say, "Did you paint a green frog?" to which he would again say, "Did you paint a green frog?" This went on for months. He wasn't painting a green frog every week for months. This is all he knew to say. Then one day, I was in the kitchen while our children were at the table playing with Play-Doh. Christopher looked at me and said, "Mommy, can you squeeze the Play-Doh?" I burst into happy tears. Christopher was almost four, and that was the first time he addressed me as Mommy. Progress!

After every sixth chelation IV, we collected Christopher's urine for eight hours and sent it to a lab for analysis. This showed what metals were pulled out of his body at that time. He had mercury across the page for months, as well as aluminum and lead. The more those metals came out, the more typical Christopher became.

He was born in September, so we had him repeat the four-year-old preschool class. He had the same teacher both years. In that second year, she told us that she was so happy to see him really enjoying school and playing with the other children. It was completely the opposite of the first year, where I was told Christopher seemed younger than the other students. The year he was five, he really made a lot of progress. Looking back, I see that chelation was huge for him.

Christopher officially lost his autism diagnosis at age six, testing out of speech and Special Ed. All his OCD behaviors were gone, his meltdowns stopped, and his motor skills were greatly improved. He was now a social kid who laughed at things that were actually funny. He had friends. Girls at school liked him. He was still somewhat of a literal thinker and would get frustrated easily with his siblings. For example, he would tell me, "Susan is lying," to which I would explain that she wasn't lying; she was just a two-year-old. Because of his literal behavior, his aggressive frustration with his siblings, and his bad dreams, we began homeopathy.

We wouldn't necessarily do the same things again with Christopher if we had to do it all over again. We would not have injected him with known neurotoxins and carcinogens for the illusion of "protection" from disease (vaccination). We also would have skipped the soy formula and BPA bottles. But even if we had done those things again and were starting over with biomed, we would have done some things differently. There are other, less invasive, cheaper ways to chelate metals than IVs. We would have never used an antibiotic or anti-fungal medication. When we started this journey of recovery, we were in panic mode. We were following the DAN! doctor's recommendations to the letter. Now that we are eight years into this, we are much more confident in making health decisions for our family. After Christopher, we had three more children, two girls and another boy. We never once thought that any of them would have autism. They are not vaccinated and never had soy formula or corn syrup. They are all healthy, happy, neurotypical children.

When Christopher was seven, we did a year of sequential homeopathy. Homeopathy was an excellent way to help Christopher's immune system get rid of injected viruses and bacteria. With sequential homeopathy, we did a timeline of life events from birth to present day. This timeline included all vaccines, antibiotics, anti-fungals, and even all those chelation IVs. Once the timeline was established, we started at present day and worked backward, clearing these out of the body. Christopher stopped being aggressively frustrated with his siblings after we cleared the HepB vaccine. He also stopped having bad dreams during this time.

I have since read that homeopathy is not great for chelating metals because there is no chelator for the metals to bind to in order to exit the body. Some may disagree, but the thought is that because there is no chelator, homeopathy just redistributes the metals. Christopher developed an oxalate issue that got progressively worse as we did this year of homeopathy. (To clarify, I am not against homeopathy. It may be that our choice of practitioners wasn't the best.)

So now we had this beautiful, funny, typical boy, a brown belt in karate, with a fantastic, sarcastic sense of humor, who had an oxalate issue. Christopher's body was producing these oxalate crystals for a reason, a protective reason. Kidney stones are 78 to 90 percent oxalic acid. Christopher doesn't have kidney stones, but has enough oxalate crystals in his urine to indicate that his liver is producing them. This could be caused by a few things, one of which is lead in the liver. For Christopher, the oxalate crystals were in his bloodstream and depositing in the soft tissue around his eyes. His eyes were red, swollen, and painful most of the time. He was miserable.

Lots of foods also contain oxalates and eating these makes the symptoms worse. For two and a half years, we were forced to put him on a low-oxalate diet. Sweet potatoes, nuts, summer squash, spinach, green beans, pinto beans, most fruits, and berries were all out. I cried for two days when I realized that Christopher needed to be on the low-oxalate diet. And it didn't even seem like it was helping! I started him on Andrew Cutler's low-dose, oral chelation protocol, added all the recommended herbs and supplements for oxalate issues, and started giving him a remedy made from his own crystals. Nothing was helping.

I then heard about and researched alkaline Kangen water. I am happy to say, after eight days on the Kangen water, Christopher's eyes were back to normal. Oxalate crystals won't be formed in an alkaline body. Christopher's body was acidic and toxic. The oral chelation was taking care of the remaining heavy metals, and the Kangen water was removing metabolic waste, yeast, and other "floaters" in the cells. We were kicking this oxalic acid to the curb!

Parents to be, or parents of babies and young children, I encourage you to research. Find out for yourself what has happened to a generation of children. Ask questions until you feel a logical answer has been given and then ask more. Above all, trust your instincts. You are the God-appointed steward of your child; not the pediatrician, not your relatives. Your parental instinct trumps any expert. Expert opinions and even current day science is subject to change. If you don't feel comfortable with your pediatrician's recommendations, don't follow them! If we had just paused and done our own research, not only about vaccines, but also about formula, corn syrup, antibiotics, and anti-fungals, we could have saved money, blood, sweat, and plenty of tears. Please, trust your instincts! I encourage all parents of newly diagnosed children to never give up. Your child's body wants to heal. It's designed to heal. Recovery is possible. My Christopher is living proof!

16

Juicy Fruit
Never Ever Give Up

W HEN I GOT PREGNANT, I ALREADY KNEW THAT I WANTED TO see a midwife, breast-feed, and avoid daycare. We had been trying to conceive for so long that I'd already been lurking on the natural parenting boards for a while. I also knew we wanted to at the very least delay vaccines, not circumcise if we had a boy, and not throw tons of antibiotics at our baby. I was prepared.

So, we had a midwife. I had exactly one ultrasound, and it was just a quickie to find the heartbeat at about ten weeks. I had no flu shot, no RhoGAM, and no amniocentesis. We were prepared.

Dominic ended up being a hospital transfer with a vaginal birth (the attending doctor had C-section paperwork done and waiting, and I'm sure he was irritated he only got to bill for a vaginal birth), because I just got too tired at forty-plus hours of labor to push him out at home. I needed a bit of a break. So there was an epidural, and I am pretty sure there were some antibiotics in my IV, but I'm fuzzy on that part. We found a pediatrician willing to hold off (after a lecture, of course) on vaccines until Dominic was two and then only give one at a time, spaced out at least by a month. I breastfed until he turned three.

And he was amazing. He was developing perfectly on schedule, and I compared notes with my fellow mommies at playdates all the time. He had friends. He was talking up a storm, climbing, laughing, and labeling. Such a little miracle. Life was full of potential.

But there was also yeast. So much yeast. He developed the worst diaper rash I'd ever seen. We were using cloth diapers, so we changed our laundry routine, stripped them, did naked time, and even tried disposables. The only thing that got rid of the rash was potty training, which he did at age two. What no one told me was that cracked and bleeding on the outside means cracked and bleeding on the inside. And cracked and bleeding in the gut means leaky gut syndrome and a crashing immune system.

The doctor once even suggested using straight corn starch on his rash. I looked it up when we got home and realized that starch feeds yeast.

When Dominic turned two, the doctor said it was time to start vaccinating per our agreement. So we started. We did one vaccine at a time, and midway through that year, he got his first (and only) MMR shot. I didn't notice anything right away as far as developmental changes, but the following February, when he turned three and we attempted to start him in a Montessori preschool, Dominic had tremendous separation anxiety. And then he brought home the flu that knocked the whole family on our backs for two weeks. After a solid week of a high fever (103), Dominic stopped speaking clearly and started babbling. And a few weeks later, even the babbling stopped.

In a matter of a month, our talking, happy, interactive three-year-old regressed before our very eyes. Eight years later, I can tell you that what happened is that the measles component of the MMR he had received seven months earlier had stayed dormant in the speech center of his brain while I breastfed him. (Presumably my immunity held it off, even though I was also vaccinated for measles instead of having them naturally.) I weaned him about a week before he started preschool. The flu virus he caught there sent a cytokine storm into his brain, which activated the measles virus cells. They then destroyed the developing myelin sheathing in his brain. It took a number of years of testing and backtracking to get to this point, and it's not something we'll ever prove. But we know.

We went to the pediatrician, who ordered speech and occupational therapies. We got a brain MRI and a sedated ABR (auditory brainstem response—a hearing test). We had our first IEP (Individualized Educational Plan) and got some Early Intervention. We found nothing. The audiologist was the first one who said the "A" word. He said, "You might need to look at autism." And I said, "But he doesn't fit the diagnostic criteria—he didn't regress until after his third birthday." We rode the denial train right out of there.

The occupational therapist we were seeing suggested that we should consider a gluten-free diet. By this point, I had made an appointment with a Defeat Autism Now! (DAN!) doctor and had our pediatrician get us into the best pediatric neurologist in town. We saw the neurologist a week before the DAN! doctor, and I will never forget what he did. He wrote these words on a prescription pad: "Autistic Regression Syndrome." He didn't even say the words or look us in the eye. He said that this was something neurologists were seeing a lot of now, and that they didn't know why. And he sent us out with just that one slip of paper. He gave us no resources, directions, or support suggestions. We came home after that appointment, and both my husband and I just sobbed. The next week, we saw the DAN! doctor and left with $1,000 worth of tests to do, supplements to start, and a very restrictive gluten-, casein- and soy-free (CFCFSF) diet that I had no idea how I was going to pull off. We had no hope. I read Jenny McCarthy's *Mother Warriors* that week, cover to cover, and sobbed my eyes out. That book put steel in my spine. If they could do it, so could we.

When we told our pediatrician about the DAN! doctor, his eyes rolled so far back in his head he resembled a Las Vegas slot machine. And he told us that gluten-free diets didn't do anything, not even for Celiac disease; that the only thing we could maybe try was ABA (applied behavior analysis) therapy, though we couldn't afford it anyway (those were his words). We never went back to him.

The GFCFSF diet the DAN! doctor put Dominic on was a miracle. In the first week, it was like watching a dark cloud lift over our son's eyes, and we started to see him again. His ATEC (Autism Treatment Evaluation Checklist, a tool used by the community to measure effectiveness of treatments) was 92. I learned how to do stool and urine collections, and we held our screaming four-year-old down for what seemed like countless vials of blood. And then the DAN! doctor fine-tuned.

Every time we visited, we spent a ton of money. Some things were good—the diet, essential fatty acids, probiotics. Some things were really bad—chelation was horrible, and in three doses of the prescription chelator oral DMPS we lost every gain we'd made since starting the DAN! protocol and then some.

I learned that the DAN! doctor would give us generally whatever we asked for. He was at that time one of the few DAN! doctors in the country who still took health insurance, so I figured we were getting a bargain. I started spending my whole lunch hour every day reading studies, taking notes, stalking the Internet—looking for that next thing that would help Dominic and then writing it down so I could tell the DAN! to prescribe it. Oh, and I started blogging, so I could keep a history of what we tried and whether it worked. By the next summer, we had raised enough money to start ABA therapy, and I bullied our health insurance company into reimbursing us for it. We did ABA fifteen hours a week for three and a half years. Some days were positive, with Dominic making good gains in areas of speech and participation in activities, but some days he struggled mightily to just be there. It was very hard to watch. It was an in-center program that is local to us, and I'm glad we did it. We learned a lot of techniques that way, too, and I really believe the support and tools the regular meetings saved our sanity. But we never stopped trying to find our answer, our missing piece, that thing that when we gave it to Dominic would magically fix all the damage. We did all the supplement fads that came through, and we constantly fought yeast. For Dominic, the yeast presented as brain fog, hyperactivity, uncomfortable bowels, and uncontrollable giggling. Basically, he was drunk off the yeast fermenting in his gut.

Fast forward to 2012. We started seeing an amazing craniosacral chiropractor in Colorado Springs who had decided that she wanted to heal autism. We have seen her weekly since then, and she can stop a yeast rage in five minutes. It was and is amazing to see my formerly completely combative child crawl in her lap and watch her place her hands on his head. Every time it floors me.

When Dominic had just turned seven and was still getting ABA therapy, I was still digging for the latest and greatest treatments that might make a difference for us. His ATEC was down to around 25 at this point from the various biomedical and therapeutic interventions we had done. Almost all the points that remained were in the speech category. He still was not communicating in more than one- or two-word phrases, and it was so exhausting and demoralizing. I just wanted to be able to have a conversation with my son. We tried multiple out-of-the-box, controversial treatments. The DAN! doctor stopped taking insurance, so we stepped out on our own. For two years, we had only our family practitioner and our chiropractor supporting us. All the protocols we did those two years were ones that I found online and had a feeling we should try. We made some progress, but Dominic yo-yoed badly. Two steps forward, one back, one forward, two back, and so on. Nothing was giving us consistent forward progress. I couldn't figure out the problem.

At the end of 2014, we started working with another provider. She is semi-local to us, an autism mom who opened up a clinic to help other families. She told us about the IonCleanse by AMD Footbaths. There are many different ionic footbaths on the market, but this one was special. It had patents, was made in the United States, and apparently no other machine out there had the safety rating this one did. The footbath purported to invoke a detoxification response. I was a huge skeptic at this point. We did one footbath treatment in the clinic, and at the time I told the provider that there was no way I could afford one.

A few months later, the Thinking Moms' Revolution coordinated a study that used the footbaths. I was convinced they were a scam; however, the attitude that I carry every day is that I refuse to look back in a decade and regret not trying something. So we committed to the study. Dominic's ATEC at the beginning of the study was a 29. After the first month, he dropped 16 points. And interesting things started happening, little signs of what was to come—he was attempting to sing, he was sitting calmly for haircuts for the first time, and he was showing an interest in and ability to play with his Wii. All these things were small glimmers of hope.

This footbath had my attention. I dropped almost everything else we were doing to focus on detoxing. I also did something that, in hindsight, was brilliant—I ran DNA tests on the whole family and we discovered that Dominic was only detoxifying about 15 percent on his own (compared to a regular person who can detoxify entirely on his own). The provider I was working with told me that if she had not already met Dominic, she'd be unsure if she could help him because his genetics were a complete mess. This was our answer to why nothing gave us continued progress. If the detox pathways are doors, his door was barely cracked open. Little stuff could get through, but the big stuff—forget it. No wonder everything we'd done to kill pathogens and manage yeast didn't move us forward. He literally couldn't excrete the resulting dead stuff, and it was stacked up, blocking the good supplements from working. It was like a light-bulb exploded over my head.

We continued to work with the clinic, and we dug into Dominic's genetics. We slowly supplemented him with good-quality (oh, they are expensive) supplements to support his methylation and detox cycles. And he continued to get better. We continued the IonCleanse by AMD footbaths at least four times a week. They have made all the other protocols we have tried since work better.

We have, at this writing, been using the IonCleanse for fifteen months. It has given me hope that we will get to full recovery. Dominic's ATEC ranges from 6-10 on any given day and has been STABLE at that level for six months. We will never be without the IonCleanse. It is our base protocol—meaning the foundation upon which we build. Without it, everything would fall.

I have realized in the last five years that the autism community is fragmented. Many people truly believe our children aren't sick—they are just quirky, and we shouldn't be trying to fix them. I cannot wrap my head around this attitude because I know full good and well Dominic *was* fine. And then he wasn't. I believe in my heart that if we had vaccinated him on schedule, he would've just never developed. We had such a clear regression because he had the opportunity to develop while we waited to vaccinate. I know my child wasn't born this way.

In these last few years, I've found the most amazing community of autism warrior sisters. I have met my best friends doing this healing work on my child. Autism moms have backbones of steel and hearts of gold. We take care of our own. I am so honored to have been asked to tell our story for this collection, because it is in the telling of our stories that we help prevent what happened to our children from happening to others.

17

Queen B
In Hindsight

W E'VE BEEN ON THIS AUTISM JOURNEY FOR EIGHT YEARS; IT'S hard to know where to begin when telling our story. I really want to share all the events that we know led to my daughter's autism diagnosis, but it would end up being more of a book than a chapter—a very long book full of heartbreak, fear, anguish, deceit, lies . . . the list could go on and on. Although it was important to experience the bad medical advice because it led us to the real truth of what happened to our daughter, on some level, I could have done without that part and skipped right to the healing. Once that understanding of the damage, done at the hands of a mainstream medical system whose job it was to protect her, really sunk in—well, you don't come out on the other end of that type of realization as the same person.

When I meet parents of a child newly diagnosed with autism, ADHD, ODD, and/or seizures, I automatically assume the "mother hen" role with them. Although I may come off as overbearing, what

I'm really trying to do is to save them from the mistakes I made. I want to shove eight years of ups and downs on this journey and my "do not do" list into one sentence. The passing of time is difficult to deal with when it comes to autism. The journey is a marathon. But as much as I hate to face it, the clock is ticking. I am sprinting as fast as I can to find the answers we need to lead my daughter to recovery, because childhood only lasts so long and I want her to be able to enjoy some of it.

It was a squelching July morning in the summer of 2005, and I was making day care plans for my four-year-old son so I could take Lily, who was almost three years old, to her daily three-hour-long therapy. She needed to go to therapy. After she was diagnosed with moderate to severe autism at twenty-five months, I needed to take her there to feel like I was doing something to help her, because I truly felt helpless. I was desperately trying to connect with my daughter and understand why she was upset all of the time.

Per usual, I was running around the house like a crazy person while my son entertained himself by watching TV and Lily sat in the corner of the room and stared at her toy elephant. She was completely disconnected from the world at almost three years old and had zero expressive or receptive language. While I was upstairs, I heard the door slam and remembered that I had not closed the outside garage door earlier in the morning when I had taken out the garbage. I'd left the door up because I knew we would be leaving later that morning to go to therapy. I wasn't in a panic yet because Lily had never attempted to open a door or even go outside. She really didn't initiate any type of activity. In fact, our biggest concern at the time was trying to engage her in the world around her, so it never occurred to me that I would need to protect her from it.

As I came into the family room, I saw my son in the same spot I had left him, but Lily was gone. I scanned the room and saw that the door to the laundry room was open, and the door that leads to the garage from the laundry room was closed. It became clear that Lily had escaped through the laundry room into the garage and out into the neighborhood, and I had no idea how long she had been gone. I questioned my four-year-old about where his sister went, as though it was his responsibility to keep track of her that day. I'm convinced this day will be etched in his mind forever; we should probably start the therapy fund now.

Standing in the driveway, I scanned the neighborhood. It became very apparent that Lily had been gone several minutes before the door slammed. Panic set in. I threw my son in the van and took off.

To say I was an incoherent mess is probably one of the biggest understatements ever made. I still remember my son begging me, "Stop screaming, Mommy! You're hurting my ears!" In those moments, as a parent, you know what the right thing to do is. I should have remained calm and collected for my son. However, the fear and anxiety had taken over, and all my good parenting sense from all of the books I'd read, which I thought helped make me such a great parent, went out the window. All I could think about was that our house sat a quarter mile east of the DuPage River.

I still think about how I must have looked that day in our usually quiet neighborhood at 10:30 a.m. driving around screaming a scream that would rival any horror movie scream—a scream that I knew deep down she wouldn't respond to even if she heard me. At that point, she didn't respond to anything and was nonverbal. And, of course, knowing this added even more to my panic.

I stopped the first car I encountered and begged a stranger to help me look for my daughter and call the police for me (my phone was dead). More screaming and praying ensued, as I continued to drive around our neighborhood, which consists of four blocks. I wanted everyone to wake up from their suburban slumber—in more ways than one. This was not how our daughter's story, our family's story, was supposed to turn out. We couldn't be the only ones who had gone through the devastation of raising a child with severe autism, could we? We were just beginning to understand that this wasn't a rare condition anymore. How could people be drinking coffee and watching *Oprah* while this was happening?

I once again came across the man who called the police, who was also helping look. He told me that he called the police, and they told him that twelve units had been deployed to find her. This wasn't just a harmless little "my child got away from me for a second" incident. The gravity of the fact that my daughter may never come home set in for me, and there no words to explain the panic and fear that took over my entire body. (If you can't go crazy when your child has gone missing, when can you?) I stopped another neighbor I barely knew to ask about Lily. He said he had seen a little girl in the street a few houses down and that it appeared she was playing with an older child. I wanted to tell him that my daughter doesn't play and doesn't really know anyone else exists. But there was no time for that now.

I drove slowly, continuing to scream and cry her name. Neighbors were coming out of their houses to see what the commotion was about. As I drove down the same block again, another officer stopped me to assure me that an entire fleet of police cars was scanning our village. I noticed another police car pull up to a home along the river.

Within a few minutes, it was over. They had found her. I guess my obvious distress was enough for them to realize that I wasn't a neglectful parent who was letting my child roam the neighborhood unsupervised. As my son and I were led to this house, it occurred to me that this was a house I passed by every day but didn't really know who lived inside. It looked like we were about to meet the resident under some interesting circumstances.

The officer informed me that the woman had called the police and brought Lily inside because she saw her playing in the street and running in circles. That's when I knew for sure we had found her. I explained that my daughter was developmentally delayed and non-verbal; in my panic, I still couldn't even say she was diagnosed with autism. It was so obvious to everyone, so why did I also need to say that ugly word that had taken so much from my daughter and my family already?

My little runaway was playing in the neighbors' toy box and didn't even realize I was there. As we were leaving, the neighbor told me she actually heard me screaming for her after she had brought her inside. She'd heard me. Don't get me wrong—I thank God for this woman every single day. However, I always wondered why she didn't wait outside, especially when she heard a mother desperately screaming for her child. Was it a little zinger she wanted to throw my way? A way for me to "pay" for my neglect? Looking back, I really can't blame her. She had no idea about our situation, and I wasn't about to have a sit-down with her to explain. I would like to say that we were lifelong friends after this incident, but I cannot. I would see her in passing, but we never spoke again.

Lily had started fading away in May 2004 when she was around nine months old. I can't give an exact day or time. That period of our lives was such a blur, and the events that led up to her fading away seem so similar to what other parents experience with their children. As a baby, Lily had thrush issues, which could possibly be traced to her first dose of HepB. According to the VIS (Vaccine Information Statement) for HepB, any person that may have a life-threatening allergy to yeast should not receive this vaccine. Since we were completely unaware of whether she was allergic at birth, and we weren't educated on the possible adverse effects, we didn't think to question this vaccine. When we performed allergy testing for her several years later, we discovered that she was in fact highly allergic to yeast. It isn't a life-threatening allergy, but it's an allergy nonetheless. There is no reason for this vaccine to be administered to newborn babies, especially when the relative risk of a child contracting this disease is extremely rare. We will never know how much being injected with a yeast-containing vaccine affected her as a newborn baby. After she received her fourth dose of the HepB vaccine at nine months, the constant state of sickness began. The ear infections and sinus infections started to run together, treated with constant dosing of one antibiotic after another. Each time the infections would come back, stronger and harder to eliminate.

The second time we noticed a pronounced regression was after Lily's flu vaccine at sixteen months. She wasn't a happy baby anymore, and she seemed to be in constant discomfort. She slipped further and further into her own world. Even though she was sick so often, the pediatrician did not once recommend delaying her vaccines. By twenty-five months, we had seen a developmental psychologist who slapped her with an autism diagnosis. The complete lack of help or guidance provided to us by this psychologist was bewildering. All the doctor could recommend was that we start ABA right away; she gave us information about an intensive behavioral program offered through Early Intervention. That was it.

When I asked about her thoughts on diet changes, she said that special diets would not help. Then I asked about the possibility of a link between vaccines and autism. With complete confidence, the doctor said vaccines had nothing to do with autism. I wasn't so confident in her answer. Even early on in the journey, something that could be called either common sense or my mommy instinct made me wonder how a doctor could be so sure about what doesn't work when they didn't even understand why my child had regressed into autism in the first place?

Do not be afraid to question your child's pediatrician about vaccines or medications they are prescribing. I was always a rule follower and looked to the pediatrician as an authority figure. It never once occurred to me to read the package insert for the vaccines they were administering, or to consider how many more vaccines they were giving my child compared to the timing and number I had received as a child. I never paused to consider the toxic ingredients the vaccines contained. If the doctor takes offense to your questioning, run away as fast as you can and find another provider.

There are more and more doctors out there who get it, so don't waste your time with doctors that don't. We learned this lesson the hard way by staying with a pediatrician's office who dismissed me as an overbearing mom when I expressed concerns about her health decline after each well-baby visit. I remember requesting Lily's medical records and being treated like it was a major imposition on their time to gather her files. I wanted to say, "Ummm . . . your practice injected my child with neurotoxin after neurotoxin in the form of vaccines. I think you can take five minutes to make the damn copies!"

As we were reading the records, it became clear to us much too late that Lily was having a reaction to almost every set of vaccinations from nine months old and beyond. We now know, based on her medical records, that she was displaying definite signs of encephalitis, which is acute inflammation of the brain (something listed right on the package insert of almost every vaccine as a possible adverse reaction).

The next time a doctor tells you they know better than you about your child, ask them if they are the ones that will have to live with the consequences of the decisions made. We all know the answer to that question.

Do not underestimate the power of sequencing traditional therapies like speech, occupational, and physical therapy with medical and biomedical interventions that address the very real comorbid medical conditions our children with autism often face. A majority of the time, these kids have complex medical conditions that include but aren't limited to Primary Immune Deficiency, PANS (Pediatric Autoimmune Neuropsychiatric Syndrome), PANDAS (Pediatric Autoimmune Neuropsychiatric Disorders associated with Streptococcal infections), mitochondrial disease, seizures, and bowel disorders. Although you won't find any of these conditions in the DSM criteria for autism, the conditions are very real, and diagnosing physicians and pediatricians are uneducated on the symptoms to look for and how these conditions can exacerbate the symptoms of autism. When Lily was diagnosed, we were told by the developmental psychologist (whom I now want to punch in the face) that traditional therapies along with behavioral therapy (ABA) were the only interventions that would help. The day we left her office, I spent hours researching the different traditional therapies available to determine where we should begin with this course of treatment. I discovered that there are many phenomenal types of therapies and therapists out there. We discovered Floortime, ABA, Discrete Trial, RDI . . . all fantastic interventions, but they would have been better applied *after* we addressed the comorbid, complex medical conditions which exacerbated her symptoms of autism. We went the therapy-only route for almost two years. What we should have been focusing on first was her comorbid medical conditions of severe bowel disorder and PANS. When your child is in a state of constant pain and discomfort due to gastrointestinal distress and inflammation, ABA drills and play-based therapy can only do so much, since they don't address the root of the problem.

By talking to other parents while attending Lily's intensive therapy classes, I'd heard about how dietary changes could make improvements in children like mine. As I was deciding whether or not to attend, I asked the director of the therapy center if she thought it was legitimate, and she went on to remind me that dietary interventions weren't helpful and were unproven, so it would be a waste of time. I didn't go based on that advice. It is another example of the misunderstanding about autism and what is contributing to an epidemic.

Thank God I started to do my research and read Karyn Seroussi's book *Unraveling the Mystery of Autism and Pervasive Developmental Disorder.* I learned that dietary intervention not only made sense, it was one of the least invasive interventions we could do to help our child. I learned that when treating autism, as with anything else, if you don't understand the reason you are doing the protocol you are doing, it's pretty likely you aren't going to stick it out.

When Lily was four, we started the gluten-, casein-, and soy-free diet, and we noticed an almost immediate improvement in awareness.

At around the same time, we began biomedical interventions with the help of a DAN! doctor, now referred to as a MAPS physician. Over the next three years, we tried anti-fungal treatments like Diflucan and grapefruit seed extract to reduce her yeast overgrowth, anti-viral therapies like Valtrex and olive leaf extract to reduce her viral load, and a bio-film protocol to help all of the above protocols work more efficiently. We did notice slight improvements in her health here and there, but tens of thousands of dollars later, her DAN! physician and we came to the conclusion that Lily's case was considered a "tough nut," and they didn't know what else to do to help.

During the course of biomedical treatment, between the ages of five and seven-and-a-half years old, Lily would go through periods where she would scream for hours on end. And I mean HOURS! We were never sure if her discomfort was due to any particular protocol she was on or if there was something else hurting her that she couldn't verbally tell us. The screaming was awful! At almost six years old, she started pulling out her hair in clumps. She almost looked like a child who had been through chemotherapy because she had completely pulled out a good portion of her hair on the top of her head. We took her to the pediatrician, ENT, dermatologist, and they all really wanted to help and get to the source of what was causing the pain. However, when they would hear the "A" word, it was as if every symptom we had discussed would suddenly fit under the autism umbrella in their mind. It was so revealing in appointment after appointment that the physicians I was seeking out to treat my child had very little knowledge of the comorbid conditions that go along with autism. They had their theories: it was behavior, sinuses, and migraines. The ENT suggested a CAT scan, which we thought may reveal an internal source for the pain, but it found nothing.

We tried acupuncture, craniosacral therapy, and lymphatic massage. Our lives were in a constant state of survival mode because we felt frozen and held hostage each day by the unknown. We weren't able to leave and were in despair because it seemed that no one knew how to help my daughter. I truly felt we had exhausted every medical option for treatment. I didn't know how much longer I could watch my child suffer and not know how to help her. It's hard to even begin to explain the anguish of watching her scream for hours and not be able to offer more than love and making her as comfortable as possible.

On the days that I sent her to school, I was always waiting for the phone to ring. Her teachers would often call and ask me to pick her up because she was so uncomfortable and they didn't know how to help. Looking back, I probably should have home schooled her during this time because I couldn't expect her teachers to address her educational needs when she was in constant pain.

I truly felt helpless and that we had exhausted all of our options. Part of me wanted to take Lily to Chicago, to one of the top children's hospitals, and just ask them, "What is wrong with my child?" I had grown so accustomed to receiving medical advice that didn't help and educating doctors on what they considered to be the mystery of autism that I couldn't go to them anymore. I was desperate, she was in pain, and our marriage was on the verge of falling apart from the constant stress. I knew that I had to do something. I had to be the one to lead the charge on her healing since it seemed that no one else knew my child but me.

By the grace of God, I came across information regarding the Specific Carbohydrate Diet on the TACA (Talk About Curing Autism) website. This is a dietary intervention strategy for children and adults that can help eliminate the symptoms of and heal conditions like ulcerative colitis and Crohn's disease. The TACA site referred me to Elaine Gotschall's book *Breaking the Vicious Cycle*, which was a comprehensive compilation of the science behind the diet. The book explains how the diet has helped so many and includes a step-by-step guide for getting started.

Based on numerous biomedical labs performed by her DAN! doctor when she was between four and seven years old, we knew that Lily had severe yeast and bacteria overgrowth. The idea behind SCD is to eliminate grains and starches from the diet and in turn she would have tremendous relief from possible gastrointestinal symptoms. This type of eating plan starves the overgrowth of pathogens in the body because they feed upon sugar and starches. In her book, Gotschall made very clear that a lot of work would be involved but, if it helped you or your child, it would be worth it. The diet involved continuously cutting and pureeing vegetables in a form that Lily would eat. Carrot fries and zucchini chips became a staple in her daily lunches. But the labor of love proved to be helping Lily which truly answered our prayers. We noticed a change right away. For starters, she stopped screaming and seemed to be more comfortable in her own skin. She was talking a little more and seemed more alert. After almost four years of biomedical and dietary interventions, we had found a treatment that didn't cost us much more than a higher grocery bill due to the abundance of fresh produce and lots of prep time. It makes me shudder to think what would have happened if we had given up searching at year two or three.

The advice I want to give: don't act like everything is okay in front of your family and friends for the sake of being strong. After the autism diagnosis, I spent so much time putting on a brave front, pretending that we were all good and didn't need anything from anyone. Yet I always wondered why family and friends weren't coming to our door with casseroles and offering childcare along with loving support and kind words of hope. They had no idea that I needed these things, because I didn't let them in on what was happening. I was so damn convincing in my "we've got this" mode. Sometimes loved ones want to help, but they don't know how. This is the time when we need to be brave enough to ask for exactly what we need.

Do not spend too much time on the people who just don't get it. You know the ones I'm talking about: the people who continue to question the validity of what we know happened to our children. Even after you provide them with the studies and the resources, they aren't ever going to be receptive if they aren't ready to have their mind completely blown by the truth. If they aren't willing to listen to your story and learn from your experience, you are wasting time and energy that could be given to your child instead. If there is anything positive to come out of our daughter's diagnosis, it's that the right people have stayed or been brought into our lives and the wrong people are no longer there. End of story.

Finally, don't buy into the theory that there is a window for your child to improve and to recover. It is never too late to start the healing process! Over the years, it has always been interesting to me that people look at our daughter and see the obvious improvements but never ask what we are doing to bring about these improvements. I guess they think that because she still has limited verbal capabilities and an autism diagnosis that she has simply grown out of the screaming and the hair pulling.

Things have not been easy. We've had financial woes, a new baby, and jobs to manage. Admittedly, we've sometimes lost our focus. Lily is ten years old now, and we are still learning the roots of her autism and the best course of treatment. She has made tremendous strides because of diet, but we've also learned that she responds very well to homeopathy, and we're extremely excited about what is to come.

In the meantime, I share our story and learn from others who do the same. We find doctors and practitioners who know what has happened to our kids and put themselves out there despite the efforts of a government and mainstream medical system that wants to continue to deny that we even exist. We are writing our own pages of healing and recovery for our children. I will never give up until Lily can look at me one day and say, "Mom, remember when I used to have autism?"

18

Shawty

The Path to Autism Recovery, Not Always Easy but Always Worth It

M Y JOURNEY WITH AUTISM RECOVERY BEGAN LIKE MANY others, I am sure. I was the model of the OCD, Type-A career woman that has become quite common in this day and age. I really thought I had it together. And so, when my husband and I decided to try for a baby, I wanted to be prepared—I read all the books, took the courses, and researched doulas and breast-feeding.

What I didn't study at all were vaccines (everyone knows they are safe, duh!) or other toxic chemicals that we accept as "normal" nowadays. While I made sure we killed every "dangerous" germ within a three-mile radius through copious use of disinfectant wipes and bleach, I didn't think twice about eating processed foods with additives or slathering my body with toxic lotions, body washes, and perfumes. I microwaved my food and had no interest in finding organic products or considering the ramifications of genetically modified foods. I look back now and cringe at how much I didn't know when I thought I knew it all.

My pregnancy had a few issues, but nothing major. However, although I wanted an intervention-free birth, I got anything but that. I didn't go into labor on my own, so my doctor was eager to induce. I had second thoughts and cancelled the first scheduled induction, but I succumbed to the second when I was one week overdue. At the time, I didn't know enough to worry about risk factors. For instance, I had no idea about the critical role cholesterol plays in activation of oxytocin receptors. Over the years, I was praised for my low cholesterol (112), and my doctors never said a word about how levels that low are actually detrimental to physical and mental functioning. A review of the literature in PubMed will show that many mental health conditions like bipolar disorder, schizophrenia, and depression are much more common in those with low cholesterol. Even strokes are more common for those with lower than optimal cholesterol.

After twenty-plus hours of Pitocin-induced labor, I stopped dilating at five centimeters and we went in for a C-section. My beautiful son came into the world screaming. Little did I know that would be the norm for us for years.

Here we deviate a bit from the typical story. My son did not regress at twelve months like many do. He had reactions to his four-month vaccinations (he received seven in one day). The effects were striking and immediate. He went from sleeping seven or eight hours per night to sleeping maybe four hours per night, no more than two at a stretch. He was screaming most of the time, both day and night. I wore him in a baby sling and vacuumed to get him to sleep, because the white noise was one of the few things that calmed him. I was assured that it was just "colic." But, of course, it was actually brain inflammation as a result of vaccinations.

It was years later that I read the vaccine package insert that listed inconsolable crying, unusual screaming, and insomnia as possible vaccine reactions. He would scream incessantly immediately following vaccines and slept very little. Just as we would get him leveled out and calmed down from the previous round of vaccinations, it would be time for more, and the cycle would start all over again. It took years for me to connect that to the vaccinations he was receiving.

Motherhood was something I prized more than life itself. I had always wanted to be a mother. And now I felt like a complete and utter failure. I had this tiny, amazing, beautiful child, and I could not provide a world in which he could feel calm, in which he could sleep. What was I doing wrong? Why couldn't I get him to stop screaming?

There were other signs that something was off. For instance, baby books were telling me that babies can feel their mother's emotions and react to them accordingly. And yet, when I sat sobbing from sheer exhaustion, my son would look up at me and giggle? Why? I knew something was wrong; I just didn't know what.

My concerns were brushed off by the pediatrician, and I was told that this behavior is "odd" or "unusual."

Very soon, these problems had serious consequences. I quit my job because I feared someone would abuse my son if we put him in daycare because of his screaming. I walked around like a zombie because of the sleep deprivation. I remember one morning my husband looked at me as I was in tears after yet another sleepless night and said, "I'm worried about you."

"You should be," I replied. When I asked our pediatrician about my son's lack of sleeping, I was brushed off: "We don't recommend giving infants anything to make them sleep, but give Tylenol if he's fussy from teething." Thanks for nothing. There was no trying to understand why he would not sleep, no looking into the underlying causes for the constant screaming. No help whatsoever was what we got from mainstream medicine.

Later, after reading Dr. William Shaw's work on the connection between the use of Tylenol and autism (as well as asthma and ADHD) in children, I would blame myself for the many bottles of infant Tylenol we used to help with the pain he so obviously was in.

By the time he was six months old, my son contracted chicken pox; he contracted it again at three years old. His immune system was not functioning the way it was supposed to. Even with his first bout of chicken pox, he never ran a fever. His gaze was not on my eyes but rather my hairline.

His other milestones were met—until it came to language development. His lack of expressive speech was inevitably what got us Early Intervention at age two and a half.

There were obvious issues in his social development. Playgroups were a joke. When we went over to someone's house, he'd stay in their kitchen cupboards looking for Tupperware lids, showing no interest in other children. He rarely acknowledged the presence of his baby sister.

He was very schedule-driven, and if we deviated, especially when it came to his nap schedule, there was hell to pay in the way of an inconsolable, fussy, screaming child. If his schedule was interrupted, it was very hard to calm him afterward, and his sleep was often disrupted for days as well. He would not sleep in the car, and anything other than his own environment caused colossal meltdowns. I mean colossal!

We became "those" parents. We would rush out of gatherings to get our child to bed on time. We declined invitations, almost afraid to step out of our house for fear of sensory overload. Even trips to the grocery store resulted in hours-long scream-fests. I had a friend tell me I was "hiding" from the world.

We tried to cope the best we could. Because of his inability to sleep very much, we modified our house. My husband made a Dutch door so that my son could not wander out of his room on the off-chance I didn't hear him wake up in the middle of the night. I learned to sleep very lightly, and the slightest noise would have me up and bolting down the hallway toward his room. Our two-story house scared me, but the Dutch door at least slowed him down. He escaped everything; baby gates were a joke. Life was stressful to say the least, and the stress took a toll on friendships and my marriage. My husband and I began to look to each other to place blame. Those were dark days for our family.

The one good thing that helped me was a very special friendship that was a source of both comfort and information. A mom I met had been an occupational therapist using DIR (Floortime) techniques before having her child. She was able to recognize very easily what I was struggling with, and she guided me through the process of navigating Early Intervention. She also opened the door to what would be an explosion of interest and knowledge when it came to food. She shared with me the opiate-like effects that both gliadin (wheat) and casein (dairy) have on the brain. She opened my eyes to the many and varied toxins, from MSG to addictive chemicals, that are added to our foods.

It was just the tip of the iceberg, but I hit the ground running, first removing dairy and then wheat (my son's favorite foods were Cheerios and graham crackers). Yes, it was hell at first, but it was so worth it after a few months when we began to see improvements in sleep and language, as well as a decrease in tantrums and meltdowns. He even began eating a wider variety of foods. That was the beginning of our journey of hope.

As a part of our state services through Early Intervention, we needed a full occupation therapy and speech evaluation for my son. I reached out to a local autism specialist at a renowned center. I was excited for my appointment and for some answers about what was going on with our son's language development, social interactions, meltdowns, and lack of sleep. But after a long drive and the stress of getting through the hours-long appointment with an infant and a toddler on the spectrum, we left dejected. We were given a diagnosis but nothing more. We were told to find a good speech therapist. The doctor also offered a prescription but would not even consider recommending enzymes for the yeast overgrowth we strongly suspected (based on behavioral symptoms like not responding to his name and giggling in the middle of the night for no reason). We had read how certain enzymes could help with intestinal yeast overgrowth, and since it's a very benign treatment protocol, we were excited to try it. But the specialist refused! Thanks for nothing! She would not speak of biomedical treatments, period.

After that disappointing appointment, I began to do more Internet research and kept hearing about a group of physicians and practitioners who were treating autism using a biomedical approach, addressing many of the common underlying medical issues in individuals with autism. I searched out a DAN! (Defeat Autism Now!) doctor in a neighboring state and attended my first DAN! conference. I was soaking up every bit of information I could get my hands on. I learned about environmental toxicity, I listened to mainstream doctors speak about their *own* journeys with autism and how it changed their ways of thinking and practice. I read research study upon research study about things like methyl B12 therapy for speech support, low-dose naltrexone therapy for immune system dysregulation, and, of course, even more information on dietary interventions that were helping many children with gut dysbiosis like my own son had. Even though I now had two children under three, every free waking moment was spent online or reading books. I was exhausted, stressed, and overwhelmed, but at the same time, a fire had been lit, and I would not stop until I made significant changes for my son, and for my whole family.

We did a full array of testing: urine, hair, blood, and stool. My child's bodily fluids traveled to more places than I did! We started piecing his puzzle together. We immediately started methyl B-12 injections to help support his methylation pathways, which often are compromised in individuals with autism. Methylation has a role in many underlying processes including melatonin production, which helps with sleep and even detoxification! The tests revealed that there was significant gut dysbiosis (microbial imbalance), widespread inflammation, and almost no natural killer cell activity. Our child had an immune system that had all but given up!

Things started clicking—like how he got chicken pox twice and how he seldom ran fevers (and how, on the rare occasion he did, his autism symptoms seemed to get better). We knew we had to help his immune system, so we started low-dose naltrexone (LDN) for immune modulation and added even more dietary interventions: low oxalate in addition to gluten and dairy free. We had many food allergies to navigate. We consulted with a nutritionist to help guide us through that maze. We tried many, many things. Some things worked really well, others didn't. We did an antiviral protocol using Valtrex. Given his history with chicken pox, I thought this might bring significant improvement; it didn't. L-Carnitine resulted in him smelling like rotting fish and contributed to the bacterial overgrowth in his gut. There were ups and downs. We saw regression, we saw progress.

We found that my son was very low in cholesterol and yet had a very high IgG allergy to eggs. We started a cholesterol supplement, which resulted in big cognitive and emotional gains. Language was finally coming along. His sensory system appeared to be able to handle more input without major meltdowns. My husband and I celebrated once we could run more than one errand in a day without issue! That was huge for our family.

Therapies started becoming more meaningful; he participated more and made progress faster once we started biomedical interventions. His anxiety was dramatically improved with supplement support. Before we added supports, putting him to bed would take hours. My husband or I would have to lie with him until he fell asleep, then creep out of the room. If we did not do this, there would be a constant interplay of him calling out for us or coming to see if we were still there. He had compulsive thoughts about us leaving him (we rarely ever left him with anyone). It took us years to resolve this by supporting his adrenals and also adding in supports for anxiety such as GABA, L-Theanine, and Inositol.

He also transitioned from the "autism" classroom to the integrated preschool class. He used to scream just walking by the integrated classroom because of the activity level, number of children, and the sensory overload, but now he spent the duration of his day there without issue. Teachers were stunned. They all had seen his extreme sensory reaction in the past, so the change was nothing short of miraculous. I shared with them that we had started a targeted biomedical approach after extensive testing, combined with dietary fine-tuning and supplementation.

Our state coordinator regularly noted how well my son was doing, saying that he was impressed with the changes. He took copious notes on the various supplements we were trying. (It is important to note, however, that this is our journey, and each child is different. We tried a lot of stuff that didn't work, and some things had negative effects. Trial and error is going to happen until someone invents that darn magic wand.)

We continued with the modified diet. We also did homeopathy. Each intervention, each piece, was a layer, peeling back as we were getting to the root issues. It took time.

He continued making progress. His language made dramatic improvements in both the expressive and receptive areas. His vocabulary was growing, and his conversations were expanding in both number of words and language complexity. Gone were the repetitious behaviors like sitting on the floor spinning Tupperware lids. He responded when his name was called.

But there were also setbacks. We would see a reemergence of that "foggy" behavior when his yeast would flare. We would see the aggressive, short-fuse behavior when Clostridia were high, and the two would "teeter-totter." So when we treated one, the other would grow to fill its spot. We had to be smarter than the bugs. By God, I was going to beat these things that had such an impact on my child's brain.

The effort paid off. We started to see a light at the end of the tunnel. Options for kindergarten loomed in front of us, and a highly academic charter school was a possibility after all! Kindergarten was the deadline I had given myself—I had to get him recovered enough by then. Looking back now, that thinking was so silly, but I wanted to make significant progress to give him the best start in school. Now I understand there is no deadline, no timeframe. Our children can and do heal at any age! The key is consistency and finding the right therapies for your individual child.

We did more work. I listened to webinars, picked other moms' brains, cornered doctors in hallways at conferences, and made it my job to learn as much as I could. That drive also opened career doorways for me in this field. I have the pleasure of working for both New Beginnings Nutritionals and The Great Plains Laboratory. I handle their social media and also work conferences for New Beginnings. I speak to other parents about our own wonderful experiences of how supplementation has played a pivotal role in my son's recovery. I have also tried to mentor, blog, and give back as much as I can along the way. I remember what it was like in the early days, staring bleakly at a computer screen, wishing someone would respond to my post already, and then being frustrated when what had worked for their child did not work for mine.

So where are we now? My son turned ten about six months ago. He wanted a Star Wars-themed party with all of his friends. Yes, he now has friends. He has play dates and loves Legos and Star Wars. He loves reading and playing basketball. He still gets speech and occupational therapy in school, but we no longer have any outside therapies.

When my son and I meet new people who have read my blog, they assume I must be speaking about a different child. They cannot accept that he had a diagnosis of autism, especially one as severe as it was. His recent report card notes a "stellar" year from his teacher. He has a great relationship with his family. The other day, while were driving home, he called my name. I turned to look and saw that he had made a heart symbol with his hands. He said, "I heart you, Mama." That's my boy!

I think back to when all I was told was to "find him a good speech therapist," and I'm glad that's not the advice we took.

What do we still see? There is some remaining anxiety, fear of failure. He does need coaching on navigating certain issues that come up with friends and, of course, there still is residual damage resulting in some learning disabilities. We keep supporting him nutritionally as much as we can to keep repairing his brain and body. But now he gets sick appropriately, his body fights off a bug, and he gets over it.

We still do a special diet. It has actually morphed into a Paleo/SCD (Specific Carbohydrate Diet) hybrid, which is working really well for him in reducing the amount of starches that break down into sugars and feed the yeast and bacteria in his gut that we have been fighting for so long. Starving the gut bugs out, so to speak, has helped reduce his gut dysbiosis. He still takes supplements. As of this writing, we managed to resolve his yeast and Clostridia overgrowth. It took seven years, but we did it. His beautiful blue eyes are clear. Moms, you know what I mean. There is no fog; there is no "out of it" look. I see *my son*, the child who was in there all along but was held down by toxins, food allergies, dysbiosis, and who knows what else. I broke him out. AND YOU CAN, TOO!

What we did is not extraordinary; others have done it too. Don't let anyone tell you otherwise. Recovery is happening, and my son is the proof. We need to stand strong in our convictions that we are a generation of parents doing what many have said is impossible. We are recovering our children and undoing the damage done to them by man. I hope my story serves to inspire fortitude. Read it when you are exhausted and your child is in his or her room screaming or giggling hysterically at nothing at 3:00 a.m. and you're at your wit's end.

Know that while you may feel alone, you are not. There are thousands of us out there, and we know what you are going through. We know the exhaustion, the frustration, the *rage* you feel at the lack of help for your child. You are not crazy, you are not a bad parent, and you are not a failure. Read my son's story and know this can be your child's story, too. Is it tough? It sure as hell is. But there is nothing more worthwhile in this world than to see your child flourish and love, be loved, laugh, connect with others, show affection, cry over hurt feelings, be alive, and *feel* emotions. The road is long, but we are beside you. Keep marching, keep reading, searching, asking, questioning, *thinking*. We are here for you; we are your sisters and brothers on this journey, and we will not stop talking until we get our children back. Each and every one of them.

And most of all, cut yourself some slack. Get off the guilt trip and quit blaming yourself. I know you are doing it. I did it. I still fall into that trap sometimes. Guilt doesn't help anyone and it doesn't move your child forward. Let it go. Move forward and don't look back except to savor the good times. Keep your eye on that prize, go with your gut, and never lose sight of what could be. Don't accept anyone's definition of your child's capabilities. Only your child will determine how far he can go—no damn test score should limit him. Roll with the punches, but don't forget to throw a few when you need to. You are your child's best advocate and savior. You know what is best, whether you think you do or not.

A few years ago, I went into my son's first grade classroom and spoke to the students about autism. We were still fairly new to our biomedical protocol, and he was being bullied in that school. It was incredibly hard to have the conversation with my son about his autism and how his brain works differently. But a few years later, he reminded me of that visit. He looked at me and said, "I used to have autism but now I don't." He can recall certain aspects of those early days. It still brings me to tears, but instead of sorrow, they are tears of joy at the future that lies ahead of my amazing, sweet, loving son!

Update

April 2016. My son is now twelve and on the brink of puberty. Since writing our chapter, we've taken his autism recovery to the next level. One major piece was the amazing gift of participating in the first TMR/IonCleanse study that used the IonCleanse footbath system to support detoxification in the body. The wonderful people at A Major Difference wanted to look at a group of children and the benefits from their detox program. We completed the starting and monthly Autism Treatment Evaluation Checklists (ATEC). My son went from a 25 in December 2014 to a 4 by April 2015. A score of anything below a 10 is considered recovered from autism. We've done other detox protocols over the years, but this one was the most effective for my son. Since doing the IonCleanse footbath, we have also been able to eliminate or reduce many supplements! I wish we'd had an IonCleanse unit from the very beginning. Supporting his detoxification pathways was a major thing for my son—IonCleanse was just that missing piece.

We've also managed to resolve his remaining food allergies and continue to heal his gut. He has even had wheat and dairy with no reactions, although we are still a strict gluten- and dairy-free household; we mainly adhere to the Paleo diet.

We are now homeschooling by choice, not need. Before homeschooling, he was released from his remaining school therapies (occupational and speech therapy). My son is involved in gymnastics and Boy Scouts, and he is loving those experiences. While shy by nature, he is mentoring a few other boys, and it makes my heart swell to see him guiding others. Some of them also have autism, and he is very aware of what that means for them. It is a bit surreal hearing him talk about taking a boy under his wing because "it is hard for him to connect with the rest of the group." Wow. You go right ahead, baby! He was recently voted to be patrol leader. I was so proud of him, and, even more importantly, he was so proud of himself.

Autism no longer dictates our life. It is no longer something we consider before we walk out the door. We can run errands, go to loud movies, and take trips with no meltdowns or sensory overloads. Life has changed so much. I can have an open conversation with my son about autism and why some things remain more challenging for him, as he still struggles with the residual damage and his body continues to heal. But those are no longer the large roadblocks. (Ask me how I feel in a year or so when we are in full-blown puberty!)

Our experiences now shall serve to motivate and give hope to others that autism really is treatable. As a result of our journey, I have cofounded a business, Real Food Mum, as a way to help others implement a real food lifestyle. Diet has helped our family in so many ways that this is a chance for me to give others the head start I wish I had all those years ago. We can change the dialogue around autism and the chronic health challenges that once were rare and now are considered normal. The revolution is happening, one child at a time.

19
Chief
Going to War and Winning

"Is suffering really necessary? Yes and no. If you had not suffered as you have, there would be no depth to you as a human being, no humility, no compassion. You would not be reading this now. Suffering cracks open the shell of ego, and then comes a point when it has served its purpose. Suffering is necessary until you realize it is unnecessary."

Eckhart Tolle

To Madison, my toughest, yet greatest, teacher: you have taught me the most valuable things a person could know. Without you, I wouldn't be a fraction of the person I am. I am forever grateful for you.

In the fall of 2002, I left my job as a registered nurse at a local hospital to become a full-time stay-at-home mom to my daughter, Madison. My pregnancy seemed uneventful, aside from the vicious morning sickness that had forced me to take a leave of absence from my job and wish for death. After that first trimester of hell, all was going very well. I was enjoying my daily Diet Cokes and fast food. I developed a strong aversion to coffee and ground beef, but I could eat Taco Bell like nobody's business. My new BFFs were Krispy Kreme doughnuts! Minus the horrible eating, however, I did everything just right. I went to all of my prenatal appointments, took my vitamins (synthetic, I'm sure), had an ultrasound or two, got a top-of-the-line baby bed and car seat, a beautiful nursery, and a new and bigger car—the works!

I was completely submerged in mainstream everything. I had no idea there was another perspective. I had no idea I was actually setting my baby up for the catastrophe that would follow. Madison was born on a Monday night, three days before my due date. Of course, I had an epidural, Stadol for pain, and an antibiotic since the amniotic sac or bag of water that surrounds the baby had been ruptured for more than twenty-four hours. Why would I not? These things are all perfectly safe. We wouldn't put them in pregnant women if they weren't, right? Oh, and Pitocin, a medication used to induce labor: a necessity to delivering a baby nowadays. After my daughter was born, she appeared healthy, and her Apgar score was good.

She latched on like a pro when I put her to my breast—one of the only smart things I ever did. We stayed in the hospital for four days so she could be treated prophylactically with antibiotics, again due to the fact that amniotic sac had been ruptured for a long period, potentially leaving her susceptible to infection. She also received a healthy dose of Thimerosal from her hepatitis B vaccine. It was important to give her the HepB at birth so that when she got home and started shooting up with dirty needles and having unprotected sex with multiple partners, she would be protected. You just can't be too careful. All in all, a great start, wouldn't you say? Geez . . .

Madison was a colicky baby. She cried a lot. She had horrible gas and would wiggle and squirm and grunt, even in her sleep. She never slept soundly her first few weeks of life, and this concerned me, knowing that infants require a lot of sleep due to their rapidly developing brains and bodies. Along with the lack of sleep and colic, she developed a rash, mostly on her face. It wasn't raised like baby acne, which is what her pediatrician said it was. This rash was macular (small and flat), and I felt certain that she was not tolerating the formula I had begun to supplement. So at six weeks, I switched her to a soy-based formula (do not roll your eyes at me if you are in the know!). Success! Her rash cleared, her gas resolved, and she began sleeping through the night. Can I get a big amen on that! Everything rolled along fairly smoothly after that, for a while anyway.

She seemed to be developing normally in all areas. I was diligent about her well-baby appointments. I never missed one, and she was fully vaccinated. Of course she was. What kind of fool doesn't vaccinate their baby? I didn't bother looking into it. It was never a thought. You vaccinate. Period. She was good on the growth chart, rolled over, sat up, babbled, smiled, and made eye contact. Perfection! At her six-month appointment, the pediatrician noticed that her head was a bit misshapen, and we were sent to a pediatric neurosurgeon to make sure her cranial sutures were not closing prematurely. She also received five vaccines for seven different illnesses at her six-month appointment. A week or so later, she began flapping her arms in a fast motion almost as if she was trying to fly. I had no clue the two were related. I didn't know why she did it. I just thought it was "her."

Cognitively, she remained intact. The appointment with the neurosurgeon went well, and we were sent to a physiatrist to determine if she would need a helmet to reshape her skull. She was diagnosed with torticollis (a shortening or contraction of the sternocleidomastoid muscle in the neck, which can result from several causes, one being a toxic brain injury) at that appointment and underwent stretching therapy to correct it. At a follow-up appointment when she was eleven months old, I commented to the doctor that she was not yet crawling. X-rays revealed developmental dysplasia of both hips, meaning the hips were not forming normally, and we were referred to a pediatric orthopedic surgeon who performed surgery to allow proper placement of her hip bones. She was placed in a body cast for twelve weeks following the surgery.

It was a few days before her surgery that she received her twelve-month vaccines, which included five live viruses. It was during this time and shortly following the surgery that she began to regress. My perfect sleeper began waking in the night and screaming. I had never heard screaming like this. It sounded as if she were being tortured. Later, I would find out that was exactly what was happening. She also stopped making eye contact, her language stopped progressing, and she became incredibly cranky.

I didn't connect the symptoms and regression with the vaccines, thinking they were related to the surgery instead. Plus, I was a wreck due to everything that was going on with her. I was scared, and worried, and so very naive. Over the next two years, things progressively got worse. Of course, we blamed everything on the body cast she had been in. Her surgeon had informed us that being in the cast would cause a delay in her development until around age three, at which point she should be caught up with her peers. By three, she was not caught up. It was becoming more obvious that something wasn't right. I had no idea what it was, and anytime I expressed concern, I was always met with a reassurance that "she's only two" or "she's barely three, and she was in that cast." I hate to confess this, but I remember telling my husband she was retarded. I didn't mean it in an ugly or degrading way. It's just that some of her characteristics reminded me of someone who was mentally retarded, and I didn't know a better way to describe what I was seeing in her.

However, she was also doing things that were advanced for her age. For instance, she could count to twenty in three different languages when she was two, but she didn't have a lot of original speech, just a handful of words. She screamed and threw fits constantly. It seemed that if I even breathed wrong, it would set her off, and all hell would break loose. You had to walk on eggshells around her.

And that was really what led me to seek help, because it wasn't like I didn't try to discipline her. It was that no form of discipline worked. It never carried over. She never learned from it.

A few weeks after she turned three, I took her to the pediatrician and expressed my concerns about her behavior and development. My instructions from the pediatrician were to read a book about strong-willed kids. So, like any good mother, I followed her advice and read the book within a few days. I didn't even get halfway through it before I knew I wasn't just dealing with a strong-willed child. The descriptions didn't fit. At this point, I felt completely lost. I had a child who was out of control behaviorally. She seemed so unhappy. Why should any three-year-old in a loving home with everything she could ever want and a family that dotes on her be unhappy?

I had just given birth to my son and had gone through a scare with a postpartum hemorrhage, I was raising my two stepsons who at the time were fifteen and eleven, and I was very active in my community with volunteer work. My plate was full, and I was exhausted. When I think back to that time, I don't know how I kept it together.

I began praying for Madison every night. After she was asleep, I would sneak in her room, lay my hands on her, and beg God to show me what was going on with her. Maybe that sounds ridiculous, but I didn't know what else to do, and no one else seemed to share my concern. If I could only figure out what I was facing, I could work on it and I could make it better for her. For all of us. I can only imagine what my other children must have been feeling. What was it like for them when she was so out of control? It seemed like forever, but without fail, I laid my hands on her and prayed for an answer every night.

It was also during this time that she received her hepatitis A series and "coincidentally" developed the most foul, horrid, green diarrhea that burned the skin off her backside. This happened about seven or eight times per day. Imagine trying to clean her up and having to rub those "burned" placed with wipes. Sometimes, her skin would be so bad, I would just try to rinse her a little with water to clean her. She absolutely could not stand her bottom being wiped, and with good reason. How would you feel if you had open sores and someone rubbed them several times a day? I can barely stand that memory. I was ignorant enough to assume it was just from her being in diapers, which is absurd, because wearing diapers does not cause diarrhea. She had also started standing in weird positions (posturing) while flapping her hands (stimming).

One night, I was in her room praying over her, and a thought popped into my mind. It was just one word, but it was so clear. That word was *autism*. I immediately got up and went to my computer to look it up. A lot of her behaviors matched. Now, most people would probably feel discouraged, angry, sad, or scared, but I felt relief. I now had a name for what I was dealing with. Shortly after that, I made another appointment with the pediatrician and discussed her behaviors and my suspicion that she had autism.

The doctor agreed and sent us to a developmental pediatrician to confirm. It took several months to get in to see that doctor, which is a whole different story. Anyone who has gone through getting their child a diagnosis knows what I mean. By the time she was officially diagnosed, we had been through three doctors. I had reported the intestinal issues to each one, and not one of them addressed it. Why? Because there was no standard of care for kids with autism, and their physical symptoms are still to this day written off as part of their so-called psychiatric disorder. This is completely unacceptable. The medical community should be ashamed of itself for allowing these children to suffer so horribly.

After she was formally diagnosed, I decided I was going to learn everything I could about autism so I could give her the very best support available. On one random day while she was at preschool, I went to a bookstore to see what they had that might help. That day, my life would forever change. That day turned everything around. That day, the most important piece of information found its way to me, and I have never looked back. As I was perusing the books, I had already found three or four I wanted, and as I was finishing up, I picked up one last book and scanned the cover. At the bottom of the cover in small print it said, "A Mother's Story of Research and Recovery." Recovery? Wait. She recovered her child? *Ohhhh, hell.* If she can, I can. I immediately checked out and took my future home with me in a plastic bag! That book was *Unraveling the Mystery of Autism and Pervasive Developmental Disorder* by Karyn Seroussi.

As I read this book, I honestly couldn't believe what I was reading: the horrid GI problems, the vaccine connection, symptoms of yeast overgrowth and antifungals, special diets, urinary peptides, et cetera. There was a ton of science, but it seemed like science fiction. Except that my child had all of the same symptoms that this mom was talking about: the painful diarrhea, the rashes, the posturing, the flapping and stimming, the tantrums, the self-limiting diet. Most of what Madison ate contained gluten and dairy. The author talked about removing gluten and dairy from the diet as some children are unable to digest these proteins. I knew I had to try it with Madison and see if it helped.

There was only one problem. I was married to a mainstream, Western medical doctor with a double board certification and a healthy dose of skepticism. And I needed to tell him that it was plausible that for whatever reason Madison had reacted adversely to her vaccines, which had potentially injured her gut, and we were too ignorant to notice, and I needed to remove the two main sources of nutrition from her diet for at least a month to see if it helped. Oh, boy.

On top of that, my youngest was eight months old, and I did not feel comfortable continuing his vaccinations until I could look into it further. I feared that this conversation was not going to go well. But it ended up turning out much better than I anticipated. Not so much regarding the vaccines—at first—but we did agree that we would give the diet a try. After all, it wasn't going to hurt her. She only ate about six foods anyway; it wasn't as if she was being properly nourished, considering that four of the six foods came from packages that listed ingredients on them that no human can pronounce, much less expect their body to assimilate into something useful. I was relieved that I had my husband's support. Plus, with all the other things I was learning, I was going to need his knowledge, training, and expertise.

I have to say that one of the biggest assets I've had is an MD at my disposal. Being a nurse has definitely helped, but my husband has that deeper knowledge and experience. (Regarding vaccines, it would not take him long, after reviewing the literature and comparing it to Madison's clinical presentation, to see my point.)

After a short time of prep, I made the switch cold turkey. I was prepared for the withdrawal symptoms I had read about in other children when you remove their "drugs," but, honestly, she adapted very well. I was worried that it meant it wasn't going to work, but I persisted. And then . . . a miracle!

It took about four weeks, and then one day it was as if she woke up. She became aware of the world around her. It's one of the most precious memories of my life. She was alert and made eye contact. Not a lot at first, but she would turn and look at you if you called her name. These diet changes had brought her back to Earth—back to me. After that, nothing was going to stop me. You cannot imagine the fire that grew within me that day. It's exactly those types of successes that motivate you, keep you searching, keep you digging, and keep you fighting. She was gluten- and casein-free for about two months before we tried anything else.

In the meantime, I had gone to speak with a DAN! (Defeat Autism Now!) doctor, and left feeling overwhelmed with everything he suggested. Some of what he suggested was cleaning up her environment and decreasing her exposures—things like water filtration, converting our pool to salt water, changing to nontoxic cleaning supplies and personal hygiene products, and so on. It seemed crazy at the time because none of this had ever been on my radar. We also had a long discussion about vaccines, and he provided scientific evidence of the damage that they do in fact cause, according to their own package inserts.

I had also been reading the Autism Research Institute website. I started Madison on Super Nu-Thera, a high vitamin B6/magnesium supplement. Yeah, that didn't go so well. I tried three different times with different forms and each time she would become irritable and throw tantrums, and we couldn't have that! Let me just say that when you have a child who throws tantrums all day, it really does a number on you, because your instinct as a parent when your child is crying is to fix it. Often when the child is ill and in pain, there is nothing you can do in that moment to comfort them. That is the most helpless feeling I have ever felt. So when they begin to get better and then they get worse and start to have tantrums multiple times again, it is distressing. You feel like you will lose your mind.

After she had evened out again, I introduced DMG (dimethylglycine, a building block for many substances in the body and an immune system enhancer that has been shown to improve speech and behavior. among other things). And . . . nothing. *Crap.* So I tried TMG (trimethylglycine, also important for synthesizing many substances in the body) instead. Two weeks later, my daughter began stringing together three- and four-word sentences. Yeah, baby! And that's how it's gone for the past seven years. Some things she does not tolerate, and with some things there is no noticeable response. But, sometimes, whatever it is helps, and you just keep building, keep working the puzzle. Eventually, we ran about every test known to man and discovered exactly where her deficiencies were and then supplement. We could also see what was there that shouldn't be (e.g., heavy metals).

I could continue and explain to you in great detail everything we have tried. I know you want me to tell you how to recover your kid. If I just tell you, you will do it. I know what you're feeling;

I wanted that too. I just wanted someone to tell me what I was not doing. There had to be a magic bullet. But there's not. I can't provide one for you. Believe me, if I could, I would spend the rest of my life passing out magic bullets. But what I can offer you is hope. Please never give up on your child. They can and will get better. I cannot guarantee you that they will make a full recovery, but what does it hurt to believe they could? At the very least, their quality of life could be improved. You will have to go to war, but you can win.

I'm not the toughest or the smartest. Sometimes my willpower is pretty much at zero. But I get up every day with the intention to help my daughter. And that's where it starts. Your belief and persistence is where it starts. Some days I'm just maintaining. That's okay. It's a process. So, here is a list of mostly everything we've done. Diet has been the biggest component to healing, but not the only thing.

Diets: Gluten-, casein-, and soy-free; removed IgG and IgE reactive foods; Specific Carbohydrate Diet (dairy-free); organically grown foods when possible.

Supplements: Numerous vitamins and minerals, DMG & TMG, Enhansa, TruFiber, RepairVite, melatonin, probiotics, essential fatty acids, colostrum, biofilm protocol, digestive enzymes, Biocidin, acetyl l-carnitine, Coenzyme Q10, taurine, glutathione (oral, topical, nebulized, IV), N-acetyl cysteine, folinic acid, aloe vera juice, neurotransmitter support (niacinomide, GabaFlo, SerotaFlo, DopaFlo, Copper-Gold-Silver), Methyl B12.

Medications: Antifungals, Valtrex, Actos, chelation (oral, topical, rectal, IV), oxytocin (nasal), LDA (low dose allergen) therapy.

Therapies: Speech therapy, occupational therapy, music therapy, applied behavior analysis, feeding therapy, social skills classes, craniosacral therapy, Berard auditory training, neurofeedback, essential oils, homeopathy, Epsom salt baths, far-infrared sauna.

It has been over seven years now since I began to heal my daughter, and I couldn't be happier to tell you that Madison is recovered from autism! She has been discharged from all services and therapies, except for a social skills class—she still has some catching up to do in that regard. Her expressive language still needs tweaking, and she struggles with comprehension at times. She was at a six on the last ATEC I completed, and three of those six were for lingering health problems. Medically, she is not fully recovered. Her gut still does not function appropriately. She has great difficulty digesting carbohydrates and starchy foods. She still carries a toxic metal burden. But I know with all my being that eventually I will find the last few pieces of the puzzle that will complete her recovery.

There is nothing more important to me than knowing that she is free. Free from a painful body, free from struggling because her brain is affected, free from every symptom of this iatrogenesis, namely vaccine injury, that is ridiculously labeled autism. Free to enjoy her life to the fullest, which is what she deserves. She did not choose this. I chose it for her in my ignorance. I have forgiven myself for that, and I choose to move on. I hope that if you feel responsible for your child's injury, you will forgive yourself, too, for not knowing. It does not serve you or your child to carry that burden.

This is my truth. I wish it weren't, but it is. I wish I could spare my daughter the pain, suffering, and struggle, and I wish I could spare myself and those who love her the heartache. But I can't. All I can do is tell her story and use it to help someone else. I want you to know that you can do this. Do not be afraid to do what you feel is right for your child. Never give in to that fear. No matter what anyone says, even if they are an expert, they are not an expert on your child. You are! Trust your instinct. Always. It's the one thing that will never fail you. It is your guidance system, and it works beautifully when you stop and listen to it.

I have heard many times over the years from experts, doctors, and scientists that some of the things I have done to heal Madison should be considered child abuse and that these things are not scientifically based. That is not truth. It's a good thing that I no longer make decisions regarding the health of my child based on what someone else thinks, regardless of their qualifications. I did that before. Lesson learned.

Now, instead, I gather information from various experts, doctors, or scientists, and then I look it up myself and learn what I can. So my decisions are never based on fear, but instead on knowledge. Also, I ask other moms. Yep. The women I have met on this journey are amazing! They have to be some of the most intelligent women in the world. I am constantly blown away by the amount of knowledge they have. Because they, too, no longer have a choice. They have to do whatever it takes to heal their child. When you have to figure that out, you get smart real quick.

You see, we are not just moms, even though some folks out there contend that we are, and that we know nothing. We are doctors, lawyers, scientists of all kinds, nurses, social workers, teachers, pharmacists, activists, writers, and corporate executives. And when you put brains like that together along with the motivation we have in healing our kids, guess what? WE. GET. SHIT. DONE. We recover our kids. We fight for our kids. And we fight for *your* kids. Because the greatest reward, the greatest feeling, aside from healing our own, is helping others heal and preventing what happened to ours from happening to yours. Now, put on your war bonnet and get to work!

20

Sunflower
Revelation Turns into Resolution

WHEN YOU BECOME A PARENT FOR THE FIRST TIME, YOU HAVE so many hopes and aspirations for your child. You research potential names and their meanings. You start thinking about the theme for their nursery, the paint color, cribs, rockers, mobiles, and toys. You read consumer reports and do exhaustive online research to find the safety rankings of the best strollers, car seats, and baby carriers. You anticipate their participating in sports, music, theater, and other creative activities. Where are the best schools, and where might they go to college? You are looking toward the far horizon with hope and confidence.

Our first son was born in 2005 and was a pure joy to our entire family. Then our second son, Ryan, was born eighteen months later in 2006, and we had all the proud expectations of parents of two boys. The future was bright. We had happy, healthy babies.

During the early years in your child's life, you are expected to attend well-baby visits. I loved the opportunity to weigh them and have their height and weight checked against the growth charts. It was exciting to see the forecast of their eventual size at adulthood. At that time, we had no reason to question the medical protocol. There was no discussion of how many vaccines were being administered to our children. We were neither provided an information sheet prior to vaccination (known as a VIS sheet) nor given the opportunity for "written and informed consent," as is required by law. When we brought forth reasonable and natural questions, the doctor and staff were always very vague in their answers and in a hurry to administer the vaccine as soon as possible. We were told firmly, "no shots, no school," and felt pressure to comply. Well, we now know that "NS-NS" is simply *not* true!

My intuition told me that something about this process and the behavior of the medical staff was wrong. Why the resistance when we ask thoughtful questions? We were not trying to cause trouble; we just wanted to know what was going on. As informed parents, shouldn't we strive to learn everything we can about the health care of our children?

Our plan was to raise the boys at home, and I intended to be a full-time, stay-at-home mom. So why in the world would the boys need a hepatitis B vaccination when they would never be exposed to either intravenous drug use or illicit sexual activity (the primary risk factors for hepatitis B)? I remember at one point, it was too painful for me to watch as one of my sons was strapped down and injected in his legs and arms at once.

I recall a nurse telling us at one point, "Oh, we decided to give Ryan more shots just to save you an office visit." Seriously?! It is *not* her place to do that to your child. We had no idea at the time what they were injecting and how many vaccines were combined in one inoculation. We discovered from a doctor who reviewed our vaccine records during the National Autism Association Conference that Ryan had received even more vaccines combined with the MMR. Other doctors, after reviewing our records, have been astounded by what was injected into Ryan. The office at the time was very sly, rushing us to initial the records *after* the visit on our way out of the office. This was later presented as "proof" of our having given informed consent.

According to Dr. Joseph M. Mercola, DO (licensed physician and surgeon), "Your doctor is legally obligated to provide you with the CDC Vaccine Information Statement (VIS) sheet and discuss the potential symptoms of side effects of the vaccination(s) you or your child receive *before* vaccination takes place. If someone giving a vaccine does not do this, it is a violation of federal law." Furthermore, the National Childhood Vaccine Injury Act of 1986 also requires doctors and other vaccine providers to:

a) Keep a permanent record of all vaccines given, including the manufacturer's name and lot number;
b) Write down serious health problems, hospitalizations, injuries, and deaths that occur after vaccination in the patient's permanent medical record; and
c) File an official report of all serious health problems, hospitalizations, injuries and deaths following vaccination to the federal Vaccine Adverse Events Reporting System (VAERS).

If a vaccine provider fails to inform, record, or report, they have violated federal law. As Mary Holland, JD, coauthor of *Vaccine Epidemic*, says, "If a person can't decide what substances are injected in their blood stream, then we don't live in a free society."

Once the boys were given their vaccines, we started to notice weird and unusual things. Our older son would cry and cry all night, and my husband would have to spend hours holding him, walking through the house, comforting and soothing him. We observed delays in his speech development along with emerging sensory issues. He constantly sought our elbow pressure on his eyes and wanted his head squeezed. We learned later that this is a sign of brain inflammation.

When the pediatric staff quizzed us regarding deficiencies in the boys' developmental milestones, we were directed to the state's Early Steps system for evaluation, where we were introduced to speech, occupational, and behavioral therapy intervention. Fortunately, as time went on, our older son showed improvement. Not so much with Ryan, who is the primary focus of this chapter.

On April 15, 2009, we were told that Ryan had autism, mild to moderate, more on the mild side. In December 2010, I was invited to an open house for a Christmas gathering. A friend said that most of her mentors would be there. I was on the edge of my seat, listening to one mom's story about her autistic son. She advised me to get my sons' vaccination records immediately. When I called in the records request, the pediatrician's staff was very vague and even stated that they do not reveal the manufacturer and lot number of the vaccines. They called me later and said they thought the records had been lost. Then they claimed they had been sent to long-term storage. It was obvious that they were engaging in delay tactics in order to stall access to our own healthcare information.

We learned later, through an unnamed source, that the doctor had been reluctant to give us the records because he was afraid that he was in trouble. His concern was not for us, but for himself and his own possible jeopardy. Our source encouraged him to cooperate and to give us what we asked for. We eventually received a package of medical record copies, but with the essential information missing. I was in tears when I saw them. Not only were there no parent signatures or initials, but the manufacturer and lot number were whited out for each vaccination. This is information to which we are entitled, and it is clear that the pediatrician went to great effort to obfuscate the data trail and to hinder our ability to seek legal recourse. Do doctors really do this? You betcha!

We set ourselves on a course of discovery, to investigate every possibility of cause and effect, in a maximum effort to understand the full scope of the problem and figure out what to do about it. We were referred to a genetic specialist in 2008 and 2009 who determined, through testing, that there were no genetic traits linking either of our sons to an inherited cause of their delays. In our case, genetics were not the root cause of the onset of autism.

We contacted the Centers for Disease Control (CDC), whose representative confirmed that our pediatrician violated federal law by not giving us any pamphlets on the vaccines our boys were receiving. Nor were we ever given any descriptive data about the components in the vaccinations and their associated risks, or the opportunity to consent to or decline the immunizations administered to either of our sons. Information was clearly withheld from us.

When I finally connected the dots in December 2010, another pediatrician pointed out to us that our younger son had received shots that were not even required for school. Hepatitis A was administered, and the rotavirus vaccine (RotaTeq) was received twice. He stated, "I never give those vaccines." It is painful to recall the many sleepless nights that our boys would cry all night—while we paced the floors with them—immediately after they received multiple vaccinations. There were many long middle-of-the-night car rides to try to help them fall asleep as their little brains struggled with the effects of inflammation. There were many episodes of projectile vomiting, frequent periods of long, blank stares as Ryan suffered silent seizures, and many spiked fevers, for which we were told to give liquid Tylenol. The painful experience of continuous diarrhea was a daily certainty. The mainstream doctors we saw later would give us neither useful direction nor hope; they merely prescribed an endless and ever-changing array of psychotropic pharmaceuticals as they appeared to be simply guessing at answers to problems they didn't understand.

I also recall being advised to have a flu shot while pregnant with Ryan, which I later found out contained 25 mg of mercury. I also had old dental fillings of mercury amalgam. I remember seeing our MAPS (Medical Academy of Pediatric Special Needs) practitioner in November 2012, and he said, "Open your mouth . . . mercury, mercury, mercury!" There is a real problem when you have all that mercury leaching into your body for all those years. These are factors contributing to a child's predisposition for adverse reactions to vaccines.

Our MAPS practitioner wanted to check our boys for an MTHFR gene mutation. I had never heard of it but discovered our youngest was positive for one of the markers, negative for the other. With certain ingredients in the vaccines, it *can* trigger autism, the MAPS practitioner explained.[1]

We do have one area of mystery that might somehow be an underlying factor. However, we will probably never be able to know if this was an actual contributor to the boys' issues. My husband had completed a full military career. Upon initial entry to boot camp, he received multiple vaccines, as did all his peers. They made him so sick that he landed in the hospital for a week. Could all these invasive compounds somehow, many years later, been passed through to our children? It's a very appropriate question and exposes an area that needs much continuing research and scrutiny. Side effects can kill you and can really disrupt your DNA.

My husband and I are completely devoted to our boys, but we never imagined how challenging parenting would become. We deliberately chose to not have amniocentesis performed; we wanted to prevent any chance of harm to our babies in utero. The consulting physician was primarily focused on determining any presence of Down syndrome. Never were we warned about autism and the possible causes thereof.

---

[1] To learn more about MTHFR, see the following websites: https://babyfoodsteps.wordpress.com/2013/03/24/snips-about-snps-mthfr/?fb_source=pubv1 and https://babyfoodsteps.wordpress.com/2012/05/14/mthfr-mito-link.

A healthcare provider should always interview the parents and consult with them about the various risks babies may face from vaccination. In 2010, we had the privilege of meeting a well-respected pediatrician who spoke about vaccines causing neurological damage, especially if given in multiple amounts at a young age. This doctor takes a more holistic approach to health care and finds out the family's medical history prior to any vaccinations. This is an incredible display of care, responsibility, and due diligence. It requires a bit more work and time.

In November 2012, the Congressional Oversight and Government Reform Full Committee Hearing called "1 in 88 Children: A Look into the Federal Response to the Rising Rates of Autism" was conducted with the stated goal to "get a clearer picture on what is being done, what questions still need to be answered and what needs exist for those children, adults and families who live with an Autism Spectrum Disorder." Many families were elated to finally hear the questions voiced for which we had waited so long:

1. Has a study ever been conducted comparing unvaccinated and vaccinated children?
    Answer: NO.
2. Has there ever been a study of the effects of multiple vaccinations?
    Answer: NO.

However . . . we discovered hope. A friend shared that she was attending the National Autism Association Conference (NAA) in November 2011. That got my attention. We attended the conference, a life-changing experience for our family. We met many autism families who all told similar stories of vaccine injury. But for the first time, I heard lecturers saying we could recover our children and there was hope. I learned about biomedical intervention, homeopathy, hyperbaric oxygen therapy, infrared saunas, diet, nutrition, and supplements, and how all these processes can help our children to recover their lives.

One of the sessions was a Q & A panel with some of the top physicians in the autism recovery field. They broke out the detail of the related conditions generally described as "autism":

a.   encephalitis (brain inflammation)
b.   gastrointestinal inflammation
c.   microflora dysfunction
d.   oxidative stress
e.   heavy metal toxicity
f.   gluten and casein intolerance, and other food allergies

In May 2012, I went to Chicago to attend the AutismOne Conference, a global forum with attendees from around the world and doctors on the front lines of autism recovery presenting information. It was refreshing to be able to speak to them about vaccine damage. God forbid you bring it up to a mainstream physician. The image of an ostrich with his head in the sand comes to mind.

We had started Ryan on a gluten- and casein-free diet in November 2011. This was initiated following direct and personal advice given to us from *the* preeminent world expert in gastroenterology and its connection to autism. (Those of you who have been at this for a while can probably figure out who I am referring to.) Ryan finally had a firm bowel movement for the first time in his life! We soon noticed his speech improving slightly, and he was eating better.

For those who are unsure about the diet or think it's too hard or too expensive to maintain, we highly encourage you to try it! We only wish that we had known about these processes years ago. What happened to our boys, particularly our younger son, is no longer unusual. It's happening every day. Our children are being robbed of their childhood. It's a horrible and tragic event that never should have happened in the first place.

Meeting so many wonderful families through the conferences and hearing the lectures lit a fire in me, and I promised my younger son that I would turn this around. I often struggle with guilt for not knowing any better then and for allowing this to happen when it all could have been easily avoided. My revelation turned into resolution. I imagine myself as a battleship, bringing out the big guns to help our little boy.

Through this journey, I was grateful to discover the Thinking Moms' Revolution. When I read their daily blogs, I was blown away by them! They were so completely relatable. Two of the Thinking Moms, Goddess and Poppy, were always there for support and help as we ventured in new areas and asked advice about doctors, nutritionists, and interventions.

I am also grateful for Rebel and Barracuda of Team TMR. Rebel told me one of the best things she ever did for her daughter was to give her electrolyzed reduced water. I was intrigued. After trying out samples of the water, I noticed immediate changes in my son's speech and potty behavior. I met Barracuda at the National Autism Association Conference in 2011. She and her husband were very knowledgeable and told me to be sure to hear a particular doctor in the morning. He was brilliant!

The most helpful things for healing my son were implementing a gluten-, casein-, and grain-free diet, alkaline ionized water, biomedical intervention, homeopathy, craniosacral therapy, chiropractic care, hyperbaric oxygen therapy, neurofeedback, essential oils, and various therapies over many years including speech therapy, occupational therapy, physical therapy, and behavior therapy.

Ryan has mastered riding a bike now, but we still use training wheels. We must hold his hand in public at all times. He will often flop down in a store because he finds that pressure of lying on his stomach on the floor very calming.

We now have a custom harness, manufactured by Children's Harnesses by Elaine, to help overcome his impulsive eloping. We have also started ABA (applied behavior analysis) therapy to help with eloping. Ryan is also participating in a therapeutic horseback riding lesson once a week to help strengthen his core muscles, as well as in an ice skating program through Gliding Stars.

Our family has been given so many angels on this journey, and I thank God for them. Our speech therapist, who worked with Ryan in 2008, accompanied me to our appointment the day he was diagnosed. Our occupational therapist was truly another angel in our life, working so hard to help in so many ways. I learned a whole new language with terms such as brushing, vestibular, and proprioceptive. They used weights, jumped on trampolines, bounced him, and rolled him on huge exercise balls to give him the input his body was seeking for calming and regulation.

Ryan is not recovered yet, but he has made huge strides in every way! Ryan's speech has blossomed recently. He is teaching himself Spanish from a children's DVD series we bought him. He can solve basic math problems in addition, subtraction, and multiplication. He is speaking in more complete sentences and asking questions. He is not stuck; we see him recovering every day. Ryan is a very loving little boy, always happy. He loves his family, and we are grateful to my in-laws who have supported us tremendously on this journey. I also turn to prayer every day for our little boy and his daily path of recovery. My promise to him is to make what was wrong right. He will inspire and surprise everyone with his achievements.

My TMR nickname, Sunflower, is in honor of my late mother who passed away in 2008. Sunflowers were her favorite flower. Sunflowers are a fiery flower. They stand strong in the sunlight and are always reaching upward. Sunflowers represent kindness, love, and strength. My mother was a very strong, kind, selfless person. I am who I am because of her.

Another mom told me that, while what happened to our children was wrong, it was all in God's plan and purpose. She cited Romans 8:28: "And we know that in all things God works for the good of those that love Him who have been called according to His purpose." I truly feel that God has put people in our life for a reason. As the saying goes, "People are put in your life as either a lesson or a blessin'."

I'll never forget my dear friend sharing her story with me while attending the AutismOne Conference in Chicago in 2012. "I used to hold a lot of anger," she said, "but I need to channel that anger into recovery." I reflect on that and my faith to see us through.

Given the opportunity, I share our story. I help educate parents and encourage them to contact the good doctors who ask questions and take a more holistic approach. I reflect on Philippians 4:13: "I can do everything through Him who gives me strength." I am now a source of guidance and encouragement to other families. Recovery is possible, and we are determined to stop at nothing less. One of the many reasons I share the Thinking Moms' Revolution book and website with so many families is to offer them hope, the hope I've found. I am taking our experience and using it to help others make informed choices—something we were never given.

21

Spark
Flicker of Hope

"I DON'T SEE AUTISM," THE DOCTOR SAID AFTER JACKIE'S REEVALUA-tion. "She is social and makes great eye contact. She is speech delayed and seems to have some developmental gaps. We can keep the diagnosis on paper for now so that she continues to get the services that she needs, because she still needs them."

We are almost there, I thought. Almost! Many of the symptoms that are known as autism have disappeared. It isn't because she never had what they label as autism—it is because of all the hard work we have done to heal those symptoms.

We chose to be proactive in her healing and recovery. Just six months before this evaluation, Jackie was waking up in the night, screaming in pain and fear. She wanted us to hold her, but when we would try she would scream even louder and push us away. We didn't know what to do and didn't know what was taking over our little girl. She would run around in circles all day long and flap her arms. We would scream her name, and she wouldn't look at us or respond. She didn't make eye contact. It was as if it would cause her pain to look us in the eyes. She had some words, but mostly she would point at what she wanted and melt down when we couldn't figure it out.

Jackie was diagnosed with autism spectrum disorder just after her third birthday. I knew before then that was probably the diagnosis she would receive. I had been searching and reading everything I could about her symptoms for almost a year before her diagnosis. Jackie is my third child, and I knew what she was experiencing and how she was developing were not normal. Although I had concerns at her second-year well-child visit, she wasn't delayed. Everything was developing as it was supposed to, I was told. I had her checked again six months later and yes, now she was delayed. We got a referral and started speech and occupational therapy immediately. Her speech development at that point just stopped, as if she was stuck. I then obtained a referral to a developmental doctor and he gave the diagnosis. Autism. I left the doctor's office with three prescriptions to try out and was told to come back in two months to see how she was doing.

I left feeling confused and angry that the only thing to do was to drug my child. I didn't blindly trust in giving medications to children and thought there had to be something else to help. I only encountered one other family going through the same thing, and they were as lost as we were. Nobody could tell me what to do when she had a meltdown, when she would just stop and start screaming uncontrollably and sometimes fall on the floor and thrash around. This wasn't because she wasn't getting her way. When the meltdown happened, it was not usually when she was trying to get something—it would just come out of nowhere. Some folks said to try to avoid any situation that might cause a meltdown, and others said she would just have to learn to deal with life's situations and that we had to take her out because she had to learn to be out in society. That was easy for others to say, as they weren't trying to handle Jackie while also handling three other kids and never knowing when the meltdown would happen or why. I was stuck in panic mode going anywhere with her, but I was not giving up. I was going to try to stay strong and keep positive.

On top of all the emotional stress she was going through, Jackie was also very sick. She projectile vomited as a baby and was late sitting up and walking. Weak stomach muscles couldn't push her stools out. We did a test to check for hearing loss, because she was not talking or responding to her name. She was constantly pulling on her ears as a baby, and we figured out she was having double ear infections that continued for over a year. None of the doctors ever mentioned that all her ear infections and vomiting could be from a food allergy or intolerance.

It wasn't until my sister recommended I talk to a woman she knew from La Leche League, a breast-feeding support group, that I found out Jackie might have a dairy allergy.

Meanwhile, I never thought to question keeping her on the vaccine schedule even when she was constantly sick and on antibiotics. I didn't know that those antibiotics were further damaging her gut. I didn't know a lot of things, and neither did the doctors who were treating her.

But I wanted answers! My research continued, and eventually I came across groups of people on Facebook and Yahoo that were using alternative methods for healing and were getting results. For the first time, I learned about different paths to healing our children. I found the hope that I was searching and yearning for. I was learning all kinds of fascinating things.

The first thing was to eliminate foods that could be causing Jackie to be sick. A friend recommended a book by Julie Matthews called *Nourishing Hope for Autism* (www.nourishinghope.com). I learned that gluten and dairy must be removed from the diet, especially if there were gastrointestinal issues. To this day, I have yet to meet a child with autism who hasn't had some type of GI issue. I have heard that these children do exist, but I have never encountered one. They are rare indeed! Even when there aren't evident gut problems, there are usually other issues not being linked to food intolerances. For instance, removing the foods also stopped my daughter's unusual meltdowns. The kind that none of the doctors, therapists, or specialists could tell me how to handle or control.

It was a long, hard road to get gluten and dairy out of her diet, but boy, am I glad that I did! Jackie stopped waking up in the night screaming and was now sleeping through the night. She was making eye contact and responding to her name. She was no longer having bouts of diarrhea. The meltdowns slowed down and then stopped altogether. Yes, all this happened just from removing dairy and gluten from her diet. But, I knew I had to do more and I wanted to do more.

She was now trying to talk in sentences, but we couldn't understand anything she was saying. Her speech therapist said it was because she had apraxia. Through talking to other moms of kids with apraxia, I learned there were supplements and various diets that could be implemented to treat it, but I did not feel comfortable giving supplements and doing treatments without the guidance of a professional. In my area, I had the choice of a MAPS (Medical Academy of Pediatric Special Needs) doctor or a naturopath who treated all types of childhood illnesses. The naturopath felt like the best place to start after reviewing her credentials online (and was much more affordable), so I called up and made an appointment.

You know the feeling when you walk in somewhere and it just feels right? I sat down with her, and we started talking and didn't stop for two hours. I left there with such a different feeling than when I had seen the developmental doctor who was supposed to be the specialist in my area for autism. I felt so empowered and full of hope. I was getting answers as to why food was causing her issues. I was given the chance to test what was in her stools and immediately start on a good-quality probiotic. Once her tests came back and we found dangerous bacteria and yeast, I was given the opportunity to treat her with a very powerful yet natural herb.

She also told me about a private school where she had done many workshops for kids on the spectrum. Jackie was in special education through the county and attended public school for just a short time. That system was a failure for us. Everyday Jackie would scream when we were taking her to school and picking her up. When I asked the teacher if I could observe my daughter in the classroom, she said they do not encourage parents to come into the classroom. This put up a red flag for me.

So I made an appointment to take a tour of the school our naturopath recommended. When I sat down and talked with the director, it felt right. She told me how she started the school after becoming frustrated while searching for schools for her own children. This school had programs like brain gym, yoga, and oral motor exercises. There were monthly meetings tracking the students' progress, and they kept a very detailed chart of the child's progress and challenges. After Jackie started, the director of the school immediately called for an IEP meeting and added services to her plan. I found out through her previous IEP that she didn't even qualify for speech services; the reason her previous school gave was that she couldn't make certain noises. For a child that is speech impaired or delayed, having these services is very important for their progress.

We still have a ways to go to total recovery, but healing continues steadily, and Jackie has lost her autism diagnosis! She still has apraxia, and we're working on recovering from that now. We are still doing a gluten- and casein-free diet, but have also removed soy and GMOs. We only eat 100 percent grass-fed beef, pasture-raised chicken and eggs, and nitrate-free bacon, sausage, and lunch meat. We try to keep sugar and processed food to a minimum. I make probiotic drinks like kefir water and root beer. All beauty and cleaning supplies we use must be organic and free of allergens. We are doing energetic healing Quantum Biofeedback (SCIO) and starting on essential oils. We also take cod liver oil, magnesium, and probiotics daily.

As Jackie healed, I started her protocol for myself and my family when I realized that we all had many of the same issues. I soon found out that my health issues were directly related to hers. After Jackie was born and I first noticed her unusual health issues, mine started as well. I was vomiting, had unusual rashes appearing on my legs, and had constant diarrhea. I was losing weight without even trying.

I had a well-respected homeopath tell me that the only cases of autism she had come across that weren't caused by vaccine damage were when the mom had taken antibiotics during pregnancy. I later learned of a certain class of antibiotics that were poisoning many people who took them. They are called fluoroquinolone antibiotics and include drugs like Cipro and Levaquin. There is now a black box warning on this class, but they are still being prescribed frequently. Among many symptoms these can cause are leaky gut and candida overgrowth. These are what I was given for a sinus infection while pregnant. I have never been the same since.

These drugs don't always cause an immediate reaction, but people can notice problems even months after taking the drugs. The reaction is what we call getting floxed, and I found a support group of other people with reactions to these antibiotics. Almost all of them now have major gut issues, candida overgrowth, depression, and neuropathy. This is why I believe Jackie had such a destroyed gut at birth. She was poisoned in the womb, and then the poisoning continued as the doctor continued to vaccinate her although she was very sick. She was also continually on antibiotics, further destroying her gut. I did an IgG test—an immunoglobulin test that measures the level of certain antibodies in the blood—and it showed she reacted strongly to dairy. I removed dairy from my diet, and I no longer had the sinus and upper respiratory infections that plagued me since I was a child.

Since Jackie had such a damaged gut at birth, she was always spitting up and hated to be on her tummy. I didn't realize that this lack of tummy time was having an impact: it caused her to crawl and walk late. She skipped over important milestones. Tummy time is critical to brain development. We are now exploring different programs to help balance her brain and build those pathways that were lost during her very early years.

I know there are people who think that all of the things that moms like me do are quackery. Most of us are under the guidance of a professional, and we only give supplements based on concrete testing. We have seen our kids directly improve as a result, and it isn't just a matter of coincidence or our kids growing out of their symptoms. When mainstream doctors start to realize how powerful food is and how dangerous toxins are, more of us moms will learn to trust them again.

Today, Jackie's main problem is that her brain has motor planning problems with her lips, jaw, and tongue needed for speech. She knows what she wants to say, but her brain has a hard time coordinating her muscle movements to say it. She is receptive to everything, but has a difficult time expressing. The awesome school that she attends is working hard with her on oral motor exercises, and she is becoming more intelligible every day. Right now, her apraxia is our biggest hurdle, but she will overcome it.

I would love to see more schools adopt the policy that Jackie's school has: kids eat only the food that the child's parent sends in. They also do not use any chemicals to clean the campus. The director insisted that she doesn't know how those chemicals are affecting developing brains. I completely agree and am so thankful I don't have to worry about my daughter being exposed to all those toxins while away from me.

It's very difficult for parents of special needs kids to keep them away from foods they are allergic or intolerant to, so birthday and holiday parties at school put an added stress on the family. Many times the parents are not told about the parties, and the child gets exposed to foods they react to or they have to be left out.

But you know what? They don't miss out on any fun. We do not need to have parties filled with sugar, dyes, and who knows what else in schools. We can have our own birthday and holiday parties.

While I did not see an immediate regression in my daughter, I do believe that vaccines did affect her in a negative way. I believe vaccines affect all of our children to some degree. I am not asking you to take my word for it; I am simply asking you to do your own research. Do not just blindly believe what mainstream doctors tell you. Many haven't done any research into vaccines or autism at all. I know this because I know many nurses and doctors who saw the negative effects and decided to do more research. I know now that my daughter should not have continued to receive vaccines while she was constantly sick and on antibiotics. (A good book for leaning about all the effects of vaccines is *Vaccine Safety Manual* by Neil Z. Miller.)

I also know that when a child is vaccine damaged, it is very difficult for the parents to get justice. The vaccine court was not built on justice. The vaccine makers have blanket immunity. They have protection and cannot be sued if one of their vaccines injures a child. To read about this, you can go to National Vaccine Information Center. You can ask to read the inserts of the vaccines before they are administered.[1] The vaccines contain not only live viruses, but also highly toxic substances such as aluminum and formaldehyde. What is the cumulative effect of these toxins that are being injected through the bloodstream (instead of entering through our mucous membranes, the way we naturally receive viruses and invaders)?

As so many have said before me, what works for my child may not work for yours. I am by no means saying every child will recover like mine has, but I do believe that no matter what the child's condition is, there is hope. They should be given that chance. I have hope that this book and all of our stories will reach out and help others find the path of healing. Keep hope alive. Your child is worth it. Don't be afraid to think way outside the box, because that is usually

---

[1] To find the inserts online, you can go to www.immunize.org. To find the National Vaccine Information Center, you can go to www.nvic.org.

where we find the most useful tools in healing. I didn't accept that my daughter was going to need medication to function in life. I don't accept that she will have a permanent speech impairment. I am choosing to be a positive force for her. I know that is something we all must do for our children.

Our children feel our energy, and the positivity in our minds and hearts affects them for the better. Many negative things happen on this journey, but I have pledged to stay positive and be a light for my daughter and for all children. When she no longer needs me to fight this hard for her, I will always be a part of this community. I am ready to fight for all our kids and keep hope alive for all involved. This is my lifelong journey.

When I have extra money, I give it to moms in need. Sometimes the most valuable thing is just talking to a mom who needs someone to listen so she can let it all out. My goal is to keep the spark alive and be a positive force in this community. We will support each other so we never burn out and can continue this battle with strength, united as one.

22

ShamROCK
I Used to Be Them

IN WRITING MY CHAPTER, I HAVE HAD TO REFLECT ON THE DARKER side of my life, and my family's life, over the last eight years. It has been hard to face, let alone to write it down for all to read. But in the midst of those dark days, there have also been incredible times of joy, and I must not forget those. Our two beautiful daughters were born, we stuck together as a family, and we came out of the dark and into the light together.

Our son, S, was diagnosed with autism the day before his fifth birthday. (He is now almost eight.) I'm not going dwell on that day. I knew it was coming. You see, it took us three years of searching in the dark to get to that point. You must wonder why he wasn't diagnosed at twelve or eighteen months, like the media tells you is possible. The reason is that he wasn't autistic at twelve or eighteen months. It happened over time. S was one of the one in forty-two boys who develop "regressive autism," or autism that takes over the child's mind and body in a matter of months or years, while the parents have no clue what the hell is going on. Some of our Thinker friends will call it "iatrogenic autism" (autism caused by vaccine injury or other unintentional assaults associated with allopathic medical intervention). I'm not totally sure if this is the case for S, but if it looks, walks, and talks like a duck, then . . . *quack quack.*

So how do I tell his story? How do I explain to friends and family, many of whom have no idea what was going on? I doubt they could begin to understand the stress on our home life, living with a child who made us feel intimidated, as if we were walking on eggshells. We rarely knew when the next tantrum or uncontrolled outburst would occur. I don't think I am in a place to tell it all in great detail right now. I want S's story to be one of hope and triumph, not one of despair, fear, and grief. I want to tell him the story when he's older and hear him say, "Mom, you're crazy. What was all the fuss about? I'm fine."

We have had S in some kind of therapy since he was two years old, and it wasn't until we discovered biomedical protocols when he was six that we saw the most improvement. The last two years of that part of our journey have been the most rewarding and also the most distressing.

The process of grieving started all over again. We had to research the reasons for his symptoms, and we realized we had been lied to by doctors we trusted. Or perhaps the doctors genuinely didn't know this part of their job, but in my opinion, that's equally abhorrent.

My son's autism stemmed from a toxic overload of his immune system. I believe that there were many things that led to my son to accumulate this toxic load (heavy metals, yeast, and poor absorption). Perhaps it began with my own health, my nauseating pregnancy, and his traumatic birth. However, we now know that a single trigger event most likely tipped his toxic barrel over, and we have been cleaning up the mess ever since. That trigger, on an already loaded gun, was five shots in one day at twelve months old. Within hours, he had a reaction (as described in the manufacturer's package inserts), and within days, he was hospitalized and had surgery to remove an infection walled off in his lymph nodes.

It was a pretty extreme reaction, but at the time it was not called that. It was called a chance happening, a mystery. They told me it was a teething reaction, that he was getting his molars! And I believed those doctors. Somehow, after a week in the hospital with my baby boy, I walked out with a sense of relief that it wasn't the vaccines that put him in there, because that would have been too much for me to understand. I believed in the vaccine theory of herd immunity, and I didn't want that belief shattered. I was extremely passionate about that stance, and I wouldn't listen to any argument against it. I had that *What to Expect* book memorized. I wanted to do what everyone else did: obey the rules.

I don't like to assign that event with this lofty accolade of triggering my son's decline because it starts the wrong conversation. There is an entire media machine out there debunking everything I have to say on that issue, so I am not going to explain it, except to say that it happened and no one can deny it. In my view, the conversation that begins with "vaccines cause autism" is the wrong conversation. I think it should begin with "autism is a medical condition, and vaccines play a key role in harming our children's natural immunity and contribute to their overall toxic burden." Actually, I think removing the label "autism" altogether would be a better start. Wipe the board clean. Call it what it is. Our kids are sick, mine was sick, that's it. We know it, the CDC knows it, and no one's doing anything about it, except the parents and a few brave advocates and doctors.

Let me point out that my children have all been fully vaccinated. My son had forty-three doses by the time he went into his Special Education self-contained kindergarten class. That's right, I continued to vaccinate him after he fell ill at twelve months. Why? Well, the doctors did such a great job of allaying my fears that this was just a mystery and a coincidence. And to be honest, I was happy with that idea because I so wanted to believe it wasn't my fault. I didn't want to blame myself for not taking better care of him when he first got sick. Was I giving him enough Tylenol for the fever? Oh yeah, Tylenol. I was told recently by a prominent scientist that Tylenol stops the process of sulphation. I now realize that sulphation enables the body to detoxify the very toxins and excipients in vaccines that are foreign to the human body. If this is not working optimally, then we have a huge problem. That sort of information was earth shattering to me and made me feel ill with guilt and regret.

I didn't want to be blamed for my son's decline. How selfish of me to think of myself, I know, but I was afraid to admit fault. Defending vaccines was part of that. I felt guilty for never asking questions and not doing my own research. At that time, I didn't even know what a package insert was. Plus, my pediatrician had a policy of only seeing patients if they followed the recommended vaccine schedule. I wanted to believe that it couldn't be the vaccines, that it must be something else. That's a tough thing to deal with when you are in denial that your child is showing signs of autism. You ask yourself, "What did I do to him? What did I do wrong when I was pregnant? Why did this happen to my son?"

Let's imagine that my son's vaccine reaction did not trigger his decline. I am still left with the fact that he had an adverse reaction within hours of receiving those shots. A reaction so severe that it got him hospitalized for a week and resulted in surgery. I feel like he should get the vaccine injury equivalent of the Purple Heart! Why? Well, he took one for the team, statistically. My kid got sick . . . so yours didn't. It's almost catchy.

So, how did we begin to get him back? That's what everyone wants to know, but won't ask openly. I get wide-eyed stares when I start that conversation. Sideways nodding, silence, no questions. It's very interesting to me. But I used to be them, so I give them all a pass. One day, they will remember our conversation and say, "OMG, that crazy autism mom was right all along." I don't want to be right. I only want the truth to come out.

It wasn't until he was six that we finally stumbled across the answers we were looking for. It is a tale of coincidence, belief, divine intervention, cosmic alliances, and whatever else you want to call it. But we finally found a way to get him back from the clutches of what they still call autism.

At this time, I was going to lots of talks on autism and thought I was getting the latest and greatest information, but I hadn't found the magic potion yet. Then I heard a lecture by a doctor who treated kids with autism and ADHD via brain integration technique (BIT). BIT was a mix of kinetic healing with acupressure based on a mix of Eastern and Western techniques, which appealed to me. It was right up my alley; it was non-invasive, not too crazy, and I wouldn't have to change his diet. You see, at this point, I had never looked into the gluten- and casein-free diets because I had chosen to listen to the sources of information that dismissed them. It was just way too much work, and I was exhausted and spent at this point. My son's autism was manifesting as severe OCD and tantrums. I had very little left to give to challenge myself even more. Even my own pediatrician said the diet was just anecdotal hearsay, so we couldn't rely on it. I wanted to hear this from him because my sole purpose was to survive, for my son to survive. Without being armed with the knowledge of why food mattered, it was easy for me to dismiss it as unimportant.

The talk had me riveted. Holy hell, you mean the brain can do *what*, now? I needed to get an appointment with this doctor! Time was not on our side, and I needed solutions. This doctor was a naturopathic doctor, and slowly (remember, I was a tough nut to crack on this holistic stuff) she began to peel away at the onion that was my child and his symptoms. It was distressing to me to learn how ignorant I was about food and how it related to the body, about GMO food, sugar, corn syrup, gluten, casein, the biology of the human body, and the gut-brain connection. And boy, was ignorance bliss.

Our new doctor was able to tell me, just by observing my son, what he needed to calm down. At this point his symptoms had diminished from what they were two years prior, but he still displayed the symptoms of severe sensory behavior (rolling on the floor, bending over chairs on his tummy), no peer interaction or reciprocal play, and angry outbursts. His ability to communicate had increased since he was a nonverbal four-year-old, but his behavior was still very unpredictable and aggressive. I was worried for the future.

She sent me home asking that I read *Healing the New Childhood Epidemics* by Dr. Kenneth Bock. When I read that book, I felt that I had come home to the truth. The book seemed to describe my child in the very first chapter. For the first time I could see it. No doctor had ever been able to do that before. Within days of S's healing with his ND, things just got better and easier. Cue choirs of angels singing.

Right away, I researched and found what I now know to be closer to the truth than I have ever known before. My son could be healed naturally. I felt late to the party. Why hadn't anyone ever told me this before? I used to believe that if there was a "cure," I would hear about it on CNN. I was glued to that channel for years. I never heard that medical testing could find out what was going on and why he was behaving the way he was. He had intestinal yeast? I felt like I'd been living under a dark rock, an incredibly noisy and stressful rock, but a dark rock nonetheless. What I was about to learn sent me into a tailspin of research, reading, and hope.

We started by adding the supplements he needed to calm his neurochemistry, reduce inflammation, and control the yeast in his intestines. Then I paid attention to what I was feeding my child. I realized I had to make drastic changes when I saw the results from biomedical testing showing what he was sensitive to and what caused his inflammation. The first thing to go was dairy, and we noticed an immediate change, and I mean immediate. He started talking more, and he was engaged and less angry. We had so much hope, I was hooked. This autism bitch wasn't going to ruin my family! I was fired up! I was taking back my child, and God help anyone who got in my way! I get it now, and if anyone tries to talk to me about awareness and blue lights again, I might lose my mind.

As my awakening continued, I joined Facebook groups for support and information (those mamas know their stuff), and for the first time, I felt a call to action for my child like I had never known before. Then I came across a post for FUA (Fuck You Autism) Friday in a group called the Thinking Moms' Revolution. What? You can say that about autism on Facebook? What? It was not negative; it was a rallying cry. These ladies were saying this in public, supporting each other, defying the odds, cheering each other on in their kids' recovery. I was so overwhelmed.

The first blog I read that first Friday was by Goddess, and the title was "Ignorant Bitch." I cried and cried while reading that, as I felt I had finally found a home with women (and one man) who were fighters and Thinkers and who weren't going to take it anymore. Getting their kids and our kids better was all they cared about. I will be forever grateful to my Facebook friend who sent me over there that day.

In the last eighteen months since I clicked "like" on TMR's page (there were only two thousand of us back then), things have changed for our family in the most amazing way. My husband got on board after reading Dr. Bock's book and never really questioned my judgment on my son's healing. He understood there was more to this thing than genetics. It was extremely important to have him support me, and thank God he did. I needed that support. My daughters were getting to know their brother for the first time and could play with him now, something they hadn't known before. We were getting healthier as a family, and we were healing.

This journey has also meant a lot of change for me personally. I found myself finally waking up and finding purpose in my life. I began researching and learning all I could about biomedical protocols, natural healing methods, and alternative therapies. It all just made so much sense. I was glued to books and the computer for a solid six months.

But I must admit it has been difficult. At first, I was distraught at the realization that I'd closed my mind to this for so long. There were some brave moms who tried to tell me about diet and supplements in the past, but I wasn't ready. They knew that. But as soon as I was, I called upon them for help. They were there without judgment. I think we all find the right answers when we are ready, and thank God those moms planted the seed in my mind early on so I could go back to it later. These are tough lessons to learn, but I am thankful I met many women to teach me how to navigate these times. My passion has sometimes caused me to be impulsive, but that's my learning curve. It is very steep and fraught with challenges.

Today, I often find myself reflecting on my life "before I knew," and I can't quite recall what I was thinking! I wasn't, that's obvious, but I do this to understand what kept me from seeing the truth so I can have compassion for others who do not yet see it. We all know that there is nothing on this Earth more important to parents than their children's welfare. It evokes a kind of visceral passion and defensive instinct that we cannot interfere with. We need to be mindful of that sacred bond and not judge or feel entitled to have an opinion about it. We should show kindness and allow peace to flow.

I do have to ask myself, though, why is it so easy for everyone else to turn away from this and not want to understand this epidemic as a threat to their children or their future grandchildren? Perhaps they don't believe it, and perhaps they don't think it will happen to their kids. They might think that just because they are aware of it, that's enough. "It can't happen to our kids. We have lit everything up blue—the Empire State Building, the Eiffel Tower, and the Sydney Harbor Bridge. It can't happen to us because of all the awareness. Surely that's enough?" Well, it isn't. Awareness isn't prevention. Awareness isn't treatment. Awareness isn't hope.

Not long after my awakening and before TMR, I joined another group of smart women whose plan is to change the world, and when you interact with minds like that, more wheels start turning than you knew you had. So yes, now my mind rarely stops thinking. And being part of Team TMR has only enhanced that. Our new way of thinking is empowering and gives us hope. This empowerment will change the course of history for our children. We are seeing leaders in this fight whose primary job is raising their kids, many of them with at least one child with ASD, but they are showing us what it means to be brave.

There are mothers who used to be in the boardrooms on Wall Street and are now on the boards of their own non-profits so that they can fight this thing head on with all they have left. They don't get paid; they just have our kids in their hearts. I have also met many fearless doctors who refuse to be silent—they fight for our kids to get the medical treatment they need and deserve. There will be a great reward for them one day, and I will be there in the crowd cheering them on.

I truly believe that passion and hope are intrinsically linked. My job is now clear: recovering my son. I finally have hope, and it can't be taken away. S has recovered so much that he no longer meets the criteria for an ASD diagnosis. He lost his "autism" classification in our school district. This is not an official get-out-of-jail-free card, but it is indicative of how far we have come. At four years old, he had scored 112; now it's a 10. We still have work to do, but he is no longer a severe case.

S is learning how to interact with his peers. He is learning about the world around him with a new curiosity that's more typical of a five- or six-year-old. He loves to ride his bike, goes to the movies, and plays "Avengers" with his sisters. He has a few friends at school. He asks questions now, like "How do you say 'how are you?' in French, Mommy?" He can write roman numerals from one to one hundred, and he taught himself! Just today, he looked into my eyes and said, "Wow Mom! I see myself in your eyes!" He was seeing his reflection, but I was seeing much more. What he said was beautiful and mean-ingful on a level he will never understand, until the day his child says the same to him. We now have a child that is present, engaged, trusting, nurtured, and loving. I used to refer to him as a tortured soul because I could never comfort him or reach him. Now I think of him as an extension of my own soul, living and loving every moment. I can finally see myself in his eyes. What a beautiful thing.

Let me finish with a story that is often used in the special needs community to console parents when they are first thrown into this unknown and scary place. It is called "Welcome to Holland," and it is written by Emily Perl Kingsley.[1] The story generally describes a scenario where someone has planned a trip to Italy, has done all the research, and is excited for the trip, but gets off the plane in Holland. They are shocked and surprised. They wanted to go to Italy, but they learn to appreciate Holland and its tulips instead. Her point: if you spend all your time upset you didn't get to go to Italy, you will miss out on all the wonderful things about Holland.

When I first heard the story, I cried, because I was grieving and it was comforting. It still comforts many people today. But right now, I'm going to call bullshit on this essay for many reasons. I think the people of Holland would be pretty pissed to know that their country was being thought of as a dumping ground for pissed off special needs tourists from America who really wanted to go to Italy for the pasta and wine. It also assumes that all families of special needs kids are going to accept this change of plan and calmly soldier on . . . in Holland!

Using this analogy to explain what it's like in my community right now, I'm with the pissed off tourists who want to go to Italy. You see, when you learn the language in Holland, spend some time there, see all the sights, and smoke some pot, you're kind of done with it. We have to move on to where we were supposed to go. We can read, learn, and reinvent the plan. We find out that there are trains and buses out of Holland, and if there aren't any available, we

---

[1] You can read it here: http://www.our-kids.org/archives/Holland.html.

can walk. One foot in front of the other will eventually get you out. I have to do this for my husband and my daughters. Our family won't be broken by this. We're going to Italy, and we will tell every person we meet along the way how we are doing it so they can follow or find their own way. If they can't walk, we will carry them.

That's the journey I want for my family. It's very hard, but what's harder is living with what they call "autism." So whatever the world says about our approach to healing our child from autism (that disorder for which there is no known cause or cure), I say, "The world is not flat, smoking does cause cancer, and Holland is not Italy."

23

Guardian
Conquering the Roller Coasters in My Son's Life

WHEN I WAS A LITTLE GIRL, I LOVED ROLLER COASTERS. WE were fortunate because we lived approximately one hour away from a gigantic theme park. My childhood best friend, Angela, and I spent many summers riding the largest roller coasters at the park. Little did I know, my love for roller coasters would be a representation of my adult life.

Mikey and I met in November 2000. We were engaged six months later. We were married thirteen months after that, and I became pregnant with twin boys three months after that. Roller coaster accurately depicts the start of our life as a family of four. Jaden and Kale were born at thirty-eight weeks' gestation via vaginal delivery after a Pitocin-induced labor. They were healthy and large for twins, weighing more than twelve pounds between the two of them. Our roller coaster was moving faster than ever, but we were holding on tight and enjoying the ride until it came to a screeching halt on January 10, 2006.

Kale was diagnosed with autism spectrum disorder and sensory processing disorder. Six months later, he was also diagnosed with apraxia. I knew it was all coming. My husband worked the midnight shift at the time and I had twin babies . . . sleep was overrated. I spent my nights on Google. I Googled "autism signs" over and over again, and I completed the checklists. I asked my family, friends, therapists in Early Intervention—*do you think Kale has autism?* It was not a surprise the day he was diagnosed. I already knew. That was the day our roller coaster jumped off the track and descended into the world of autism. Our daily life schedule of therapy appointments and doctor appointments would then become our normal routine.

For four overlapping years of biomedical protocols, six years of dietary restrictions, two years of homeopathy, and six years of traditional therapies, our roller coaster stayed derailed. Jaden and Kale were now ten years old. How did that happen? They can't be ten years old! Kale is too old to recover from autism at ten years old! We missed the "window!" (Many professionals will often refer to the "window" of opportunity when discussing developmental milestones with a parent of a child with autism. Over and over again we were told that the best opportunity to see Kale progress in development had to happen before he turned seven years old, or progress would be harder to achieve, if it was possible at all.) Now what would we do?

My hope of him recovering from autism waivered as I thought about the years and years we worked toward recovery without making it to the other side. I fought with myself daily and focused on hope because I refused to let despair take over. I refused to give up on my son just because we had not found the right protocol or the right therapy before his tenth birthday. I knew it was out there. I just needed to research more. So, I did. I spent hours upon hours on Google again. Social media did not exist back when Kale was diagnosed. That's right, people, there was no Facebook! We had Yahoo groups, and I joined many of them.

One night just after my boys had turned ten, I was lying in bed reading through my emails. For some reason, I clicked on one of them, and that became the night our roller coaster got back on track. I read a feed in that email about homotoxicology. I was immediately intrigued and I went to Google. I learned that homotoxicology was developed by Dr. Hans-Heinrick Reckeweg and that it used homeopathic remedies that worked at both the intracellular and extracellular levels. This treatment would get the inflammation down, address the overburden/toxicity of the organs, and detox my son. Homotoxicology remedies work to open up the detox pathways in the body, pushing the toxins out. There were different phases of homotoxicology, and I remember wondering when we started the protocol which phase Kale was in.

Homotoxicology gave me that feeling almost immediately. You know the feeling I am describing—the one when you are reading and researching a protocol, and that mommy instinct kicks in, and next thing you know you are talking to your computer, screaming, "Yes, that's totally my son!"

I called that next week and made an appointment. Homotoxicology would be our focus for the next twelve months. We started the protocol in late August 2012. From the start, I knew it would be life-changing for all of us. Regardless of Kale's age, my hope, strength, and focus were renewed, and onward we went. After two months of treatment, I noticed increased eye contact, moments of pure clarity where he would look at us with those gigantic brown eyes as if he were seeing us in a different way; he was also more compliant, and he was laughing appropriately. Kale also had some huge emotional ups and downs during those first two months on the homotoxicology protocol. We even had a short return of some old behaviors, but they quickly faded again. According to our homeopath, Kale was a great responder.

The first holiday during our homotox journey was Thanksgiving. I wasn't sure what to expect because everything was still so new. We were still learning about the remedies and the way that the body detoxes. I have had anxiety around every single holiday since Kale was diagnosed with autism. So many people are around during the holidays—people who are not used to your everyday routine with a child with autism. There are also the dreaded food tables within reach of my son, who could never eat any of it because of his dietary restrictions. What kind of meltdowns was that going to cause that holiday? Would he play with the other kids or stay in his own world while we were supposed to be "visiting" with friends and family? Would he break something at my aunt's house? These questions build the anxiety within parents of children with autism around the holidays.

This particular Thanksgiving was at my brother and sister-in-law's new house. I had anxiety because it was not at my parents' house, where we know Kale is comfortable. I went with the flow of the plans, and I was blown away. That Thanksgiving, Kale sat at the dinner table, surrounded by Mikey and me, Jaden, and my parents. He sat at the dinner table and ate Thanksgiving dinner with us. That was a first in our history of holidays. He had never sat at the table and enjoyed a holiday meal with us. I took pictures. I cried. My husband cried and my parents joined in. We were in complete amazement, and we enjoyed every single second of it. My sister-in-law walked over to the table and I said, "Look at him." We smiled and enjoyed the moment. My anxiety dissipated. That was a Thanksgiving to remember. We had conquered that ride and it was amazing!

Next ride . . . Christmas, my favorite time of the year. Many Christmas celebrations have been ruined due to my anxiety and the failure of the day to live up to the picture-perfect vision of what these holidays should be. We've had many good or mediocre Christmases, but we were yet to have a Christmas where my anxiety didn't get the best of me. I usually ended up crying for one reason or another. For example, during Christmas of 2011, Kale didn't even want to open his presents. I cried the entire morning.

Our holiday typically begins on Christmas Eve with my in-laws coming over, having dinner, and opening gifts with the boys. This year, Kale was in a perky mood all day. My anxiety, although present, was at an all-time low. I think this was in part because Kale was in a good place all day, smiling and laughing with Jaden. My in-laws arrived, we ate dinner, and it was time for presents. Kale was all about opening presents that night. He wanted more, more, more. He was interested in what the gifts were, he said "thank you," and he smiled a lot. It was breathtaking, literally. Mikey and I had tears in our eyes as we watched it all unfold. We tucked him into bed that night, with his brand new weighted sleeping bag, and we felt blessed. We were thankful for those moments together, witnessed by others, that our son was truly excited for Christmas to be here.

Christmas morning arrived, and Jaden came running into our room at the crack of dawn. Kale was also awake. They both looked over the railing and smiled. They saw their piles of presents and couldn't wait to get down the stairs. Kale and Jaden descended the stairs together and ran into the family room. Side by side, they sat on the couch while I grabbed for my morning caffeine and gathered my camera to capture every single second of this most special morning. The whole time I was wondering, *is this gonna be it?* Is this finally going to be my picture-perfect holiday . . . my favorite ride in the park?

I watched in amazement that morning, as my twin babies sat together, opening their Christmas gifts from Santa. It was a ride I hope all my autism mama friends experience with their children. It was that perfect. Once again, Mikey and I cried tears of joy. We had waited a long time to experience this type of typical holiday together. We were elated.

The day continued with an annual get-together at my aunt and uncle's house for Christmas brunch. Kale continued to have a great day. Jaden confided in me that he had noticed how well his brother was doing and that it made him happy, too. When it was time for opening gifts, Kale sat in the middle of the large, over-crowded family room and waited for his gifts to be passed to him. He looked at me for approval and then tore into them. He smiled, he giggled, and he opened gifts. When he was done, with my prompts he went around the room and thanked his family members for their gifts.

The day concluded at my parents' house, where we celebrated with my brothers and their beautiful families. It had already been a long day, and Kale had already given us such happiness throughout the earlier hours of the day that I really didn't have high expectations for him to be so engaged for the remainder of our time at the autism theme park that day. I stopped and caught my breath for a moment, realizing I had no anxiety in that second. The anxiety that had been my partner during all holiday functions for so many years had left me solo to truly experience the moments of this holiday. Gladly, I was on my own for this one.

Kale surprised us once again and sat on the floor, amongst his brother and his cousins, and he opened his gifts. My mom was beaming. She was staring at him intently, with tears in her eyes. We knew in that moment that he was coming back to us. Mikey and I packed up the kids' haul from the day and we headed home. We got in the house and couldn't believe we had just experienced this day. We had just experienced the most picture-perfect family holiday I could have ever dreamt up. I would forever cherish every moment of those twenty-four hours in my heart. I was grateful, but most of all, I was excited for what the year of homotoxicology had in store for us.

Next ride: Easter bunny. We had now been doing homotoxicology for approximately seven months. I was learning so much every day. I was introduced to so many different brands of remedies. Additionally, I had a tight lock on understanding how Kale's body responded to most of the remedies and most of the brands, and I knew how to support him during detox. Things were moving along. We were having more good days than bad, although any time a child is going through detox like this, you are going to have some hard days. There can be emotional days where your child is crying for no apparent reason. There can be days full of detox behaviors, like aggression towards self or others. There can be days where they have a fever because they are pushing out a virus that has laid dormant in the organs for years. This is why it is essential to know your child's body and how to support them during the process while working closely alongside your practitioner.

Coloring eggs is a tradition that Jaden *loves*; he usually ended up doing it with just me because Kale wasn't really interested. This year, Kale sat and colored Easter eggs with his brother—independently. He didn't need me to help him dunk the eggs. He had it down. All by himself, he had it under control. He woke up on Easter morning, ran down the stairs with his brother once again, and they dove into inspecting their baskets. He smiled and giggled as he explored the contents of his basket. Again, I grabbed the camera, documented the moments both on film and in my heart, and we went about the day.

Homotoxicology was bringing him back to us. He was improving right before our eyes. His sensory aversions were dwindling and it was an amazing sight to see. He could now sit in a chair and get his hair cut. He didn't need Mikey and me to hold him down. Mikey didn't have scratches on his arms, and I didn't have hair clippings all over me from holding him during the haircut. I grabbed the camera again and I videotaped the monumental moments that just kept happening. Ten-year-old "window?" Kids cannot recover from autism once they reach a certain age? Nonsense. My son was fighting through right before my eyes and I was documenting his every moment. Our roller coaster was picking up speed, and we were headed into the corkscrew turns.

Mother's Day 2013 was a colossal moment for our family. For years, we didn't go out to dinner like typical families for many reasons—dietary restrictions, sensory overload, difficulties with waiting for long time periods, to name a few. I often found that if a situation created more anxiety than was already apparent in our everyday lives,

I respectfully declined offers and we stayed home. This Mother's Day was different. All I wanted was to go out to eat with Mikey and the boys. I felt like Kale's progress was at a point where he could handle going out to dinner if we let him have a dietary infraction. Mikey said, "Okay, if you are ready, let's do it."

We headed out that day in the early afternoon. My plan was to arrive at the family-friendly restaurant early enough so that there wasn't a long wait time for a table. We lucked out because there was no wait time at all. We were taken to a table immediately. Kale grabbed a menu and began to look it over. I am not going to lie—my anxiety came to the restaurant with us. I was nervous. What was I thinking? Was this a good idea? Finally, I had to get a grip and order our food. Kale pointed to what he wanted in the menu and then proceeded to try to push me out of the booth as if he were telling me, "Okay, Mom, I told you what I wanted, now go get it." I looked at Mikey and said, "Wow, we have to teach him that the server will bring him his food, not Mama."

We lucked out again and had an amazing server that day. Everything came out really fast and we had everything we needed. While we were at the restaurant, waiting for our food, Kale and Jaden colored on the kid's menus, played tic-tac-toe with us, and all was perfect on this ride, for that moment. Our food came, and Kale was so excited. He ate his dinner, and I remember thinking to myself how well behaved he was in those moments. Except for the fact that Kale had very little expressive speech, I really don't think anyone in that restaurant would have realized that he was a child with autism.

My Mother's Day was perfect. Again, I had tears, I took pictures, and I keep those memories in my heart. That was the best Mother's Day I had had since my beautiful twin boys were born ten years ago. It was everything I had envisioned it would be, going out to dinner as a family. We continue to take the boys out to eat once a month. This does nothing for their healthy diets, but it does wonders for the memories we are making as a family, and that trumps dietary restrictions one time a month. Kale continues to do well when we go out to eat. We have learned that he can control his verbal stimming when we are out, which is something we had no idea he could do.

It was exciting to watch Kale interact with peers his age at summer parties with the neighbors. He jumped on the big trampoline with the other kids, he swam with the other kids, and he laughed and enjoyed being the center of attention. It was the best summer of his life. It was a summer filled with roller coaster rides—the fast ones. The ones that flip, turn, and descend into the corkscrews that life throws us. It continued to be a summer of firsts for our boy. He rode his big wheel around the entire block, chasing his brother on his bike, for the first time ever. He played baseball with a bat and a tee in the backyard with his brother. He spent time at the beach with friends and he was showing us exactly how he wanted to spend his summer days.

Homotoxicology gave us our son back. With our homotox protocol, he was more engaged, more connected overall. His receptive language skills were improving. He would come downstairs to see what I wanted when I called his name from the staircase landing. He looked at us with meaning in his eyes. He no longer had to carry around a stack of animal or sight word flashcards that was ten inches thick. He didn't need to be on the iPad every minute of the day, stimming on his movies. He wanted to play with Jaden. He sat and played simple board games with me. His need to regulate his sensory system was diminishing, and he was controlling his own sensory regulation in more age-appropriate manner. He was identifying when his body needed to be regulated, and he did it by means of swinging on his sensory swings in the basement or out on the swingset or grabbing some of his sensory fidgets. He was controlling his verbal stims in public (verbal outbursts of babbling and noises that are not always words, more like verbal noises). This was all so amazing and overwhelming at the same time. We were on the right roller coaster, finally. All those years, and we finally found our favorite ride at the theme park called autism. We were on that ride and we were screaming at the top of our lungs, hands in the air!

During this time, we also did seven months of sublingual immunotherapy. This therapy allowed us to test Kale and remove the foods from his diet that were causing inflammation in his body. This protocol, in conjunction with homotoxicology, was miraculous as well. Sublingual immunotherapy taught me even more about my son's body and the foods that were safe for my son to eat. I was grocery shopping and cooking more than I ever had before. Admittedly, I am no Suzy Homemaker. However, I enjoyed it because my kids were eating exactly what their bodies needed to heal. The inflammation decreased, and I am forever changed because of that protocol. It required hours and hours of cooking on Sundays and prepping food for the week, but I learned so much.

Our journey through autism continues. Although Kale has made remarkable progress over the last twelve months, we still have a lot of rides to conquer in our theme park. Apraxia is located in the northern area of the autism theme park. It's the biggest ride in the park. It's the ride that you can see from a mile away. You know when you are driving on the highway and you are almost at the park, and that first roller coaster track appears through the trees in the skyline? Yeah, that ride! We have gotten close to riding it, but something always gets in our way and we just haven't been able to tackle that ride yet. Well, this year, it will happen. This ride has one of those really steep inclines that needs to be climbed . . . *click, click, click.* With the right harness and lap belt, it can be done. I know in my heart that we will defeat that incline, and after that . . . we will sit back and enjoy the ride.

Apraxia is our biggest struggle for Kale. Apraxia is a motor planning problem where the brain is not properly communicating with the mouth to get the words out. A lot of times kids who have apraxia will get a word out and you will rejoice, but it will be months before you hear that word again. No protocol has touched it. Therapy has been rough. Apraxia tries to take over my hope and bring me down. My response? To hell with you, apraxia! I am sick to death of you controlling my son and keeping us from full healing. No more! You may have a tight grip on my son for now, but I am coming after you this year. I can hear Kale's amazing voice in my dreams. Soon, that will be a reality. Positive affirmation is a powerful being, and it's in our house, everywhere. It will happen. Jaden asked me a few months ago, "Mom, why can Kale get his words out sometimes and then others he just can't?" I explained to Jaden that it was the apraxia and that mama was fighting it hard this year. Lots of changes on the forefront for our family this year so that I can make sure we get in line for that last ride in the theme park and that I find a way for us to successfully climb that incline on that ride. Hope remains a constant in our family. I won't let the negative in. We will get over every last hill on those roller coasters, and we will do it together.

One of the most significant happenings within the last twelve months has been the relationships that I have formed with some remarkable autism mama warriors. I am blessed to have the support of many who are fighting the same fight, who are stuck on the same roller coaster, who have conquered every ride in the theme park. I am supported, I am loved, and I am honored by these women I call my autism family. The relationships that are built upon this journey are life-changing. Without the support of these warrior mamas in my life, I would not have the knowledge, strength, and determination to wait in line and conquer every single ride in that theme park.

My fellow homotox moms know who they are. They saved me at a time when I needed saving. I am a strong autism mom. I support, love, and guide many families on this journey. Homotoxicology also brought me to the Thinking Moms' Revolution, where I was able to get to know a number of these amazing moms and dads. Additionally, I have a support system of warrior moms right here in my hometown. They, too, give me the unconditional love and support that is needed for this journey. My family, my very large family,

Mikey's family, my best friend, Katherine, and my other friends continue to be there for us every day and are our biggest supporters.

My childhood best friend, Angela, and I are still riding those coasters together in this autism theme park because she is Kale's godmother. Little did we know how our love of roller coasters would be so significant in our adult lives. All those nights spent walking the paved paths of the theme park are now spent in my kitchen, discussing our kids and their healing. Daily, we share with everyone our stories of triumph from the autism theme park. My parents, there are no words for how much they love and support us throughout this journey. I love you deeply, Mama and Daddy. To my Mikey . . . I can never say in words how grateful I am that you chose me. I only hope that you are proud of me and the work that I do and how hard I fight for our sons. I could not do any of this without you by my side. You are a true example of a warrior dad. You are among the best of them.

My hope for all of you reading this is that you find the support system needed to get through all of the lines in your theme park, on your roller coasters, and on your journey through that "window." Conquer every ride. If you haven't yet, you will, just like we will. Until then, hope will keep you going.

24

Creole Queen
I'm in Repair

"SINCE THE LORD IS DIRECTING OUR STEPS, DON'T TRY TO FIGURE out everything that happens along the way." Proverbs 20:24 tells us to trust in Him. My faith is everything to me, and when things happen, no matter what, I choose to be happy. My advice is to have patience with everything unresolved in your life. We women have to be strong. There is really no other choice.

My story is no different from that of any parent when their child is diagnosed with autism. Your heart drops, you're confused, you're going through your whole pregnancy in your mind. "What happened? How? Why?" You're asking the doctor, but he cannot tell you how it happened, or why. Okay, breathe. Let's go. Our goal is recovery.

What is recovery? According to the dictionary, it's an act or process of becoming healthy after an illness or injury. The act or process of returning to a normal state after a period of difficulty. Your recovery may be different from another's recovery. Through trial and error and research, you can eliminate the things that didn't work for your child and put your time and energy into what *does* work for your child. On the path to autism recovery, remember—you're the expert. You know your child better than anyone else. Follow that gut feeling, ask questions until you understand. Research, research, research; and with patience, prayer, and repetition, recovery can happen.

At the age of twenty-seven, I was told by my doctor it would be impossible for me to have babies. Can you imagine that? Near thirty, wanting to have kids, being told it couldn't happen. We talked about IVF and adoption. I couldn't believe I was having this conversation. A couple of years later, at the age of twenty-nine, I discovered I was pregnant. I couldn't believe it! I guess the doctor was wrong. I remember that day like it was yesterday.

My adorable baby boy was born in February 2008. Full term. Healthy. I remember holding him in my arms for the first time. Oh, my goodness! He was beautiful! Gorgeous blue eyes, nice round head, just handsome. I stayed in the hospital for three days. He cried. But that's what babies do—they cry. I was a first-time mom, so that's what I expected. I didn't see anything wrong. No sleep, who cares? He didn't want me to leave him. He wanted to be near me at all times. I didn't focus on that. I was just enjoying my beautiful baby boy.

I didn't ask questions until he was a month old. When he cried, he wouldn't allow me to cuddle him to comfort him. I had to figure out what position he wanted me to hold him in by going through multiple holding positions. I would go through the steps of making my baby happy. I checked his diaper to make sure it was clean, I patted him on the back to burp him, I timed his feeding to make sure he was fed and full. Oh, I was doing all of it. I didn't care what I had to do. I enjoyed being a mother, but it made me sad that he would cry so much and that it took a lot to comfort him.

I took him to the doctor. I was told it was colic and bad gas. I was given a colic medicine to soothe his stomach. Oh, it would make him fart, but my poor baby would still cry. As time went by, I noticed he would not allow anyone but me to hold him. He would not sleep in his bassinet or crib. He slept by me every night. If I had to take a bath, he had to be near me and see me. Later, I noticed he did not want to be in a crowd of people. I'd always had get-togethers in my home, but that completely stopped because he would cry the whole time others were there. I did not know what was going on.

We purchased so many baby things: a bassinet, a crib, a play set, and so many toys. He didn't want to sleep in his bassinet or the crib. He didn't want to play with almost any of his toys. Momma was his entertainment. I would sing the ABC song, "Twinkle, Twinkle, Little Star," and talk about anything that would keep his attention and make him happy.

I got no sleep. As a first-time mom, I thought that was normal. I was still excited that God blessed me with a baby boy. Sleep will come later, I thought. He just cried a little bit more than other babies. I stayed positive. I memorized the things he did not like. I knew he didn't like crowds of people, loud noises, certain textures, certain sounds, and riding in the car.

I went through this journey with his pediatrician. I was concerned when I noticed he wasn't talking a lot. He was one and a half at the time. We went through questions and an evaluation, and the pediatrician said some kids take a little bit more time. At two, she put in a referral to Early Steps. I remember the first visit—it was the first time I heard the word *autism*.

The service coordinator noticed that my son was playing with his ABC toy by himself. He never looked up to say hello. He never acknowledged that she was in the room. He continued to play with this toy. She called his name: "Brian." He didn't respond. She called again. No response. Now, Brian did respond to his name in those days, but only if mom or dad was calling him. So, she kneeled down to be on the same eye level as him. She asked if could she see his toy, he said "No." He started to talk to her without looking in her eyes.

During that visit, she said, "Mrs. Hertzock, I'm concerned your child is showing signs of autism." I asked her, "What is autism?" She responded, "Difficulty with verbal communication, using and understanding language, difficulty with social interaction, difficulty changing routines, repetitive body language, doesn't make eye contact, doesn't smile when smiled at, doesn't respond to his or her name, doesn't wave goodbye or point, doesn't initiate or respond to cuddling, does not like to play with other people, cannot make basic requests." The list went on and on.

As she was talking, I checked my list of the things he didn't like. "Oh, my baby," was all I could say. I couldn't believe it. She advised me to see a neurologist and a psychologist. I have to add that during this visit, I also had my one-year-old there. Yes, I became pregnant again when Brian was six months old. I began to notice these same signs with my second child.

As a baby, my second-born didn't really cry. We had to check on him constantly because he was so quiet. My major concern was that he wouldn't eat. I tried to feed him baby food at six months, but he didn't want to eat it. I took him to the doctor. They didn't find anything unusual and suggested we give it some time. Months later, he was still not eating and not speaking. He only said "mama" and "dada."

I had no idea what to do. I was puzzled. I didn't picture my second child having autism, but what parent does? I knew this wasn't the time to stop and ask why, as my kids needed me. I needed to learn what to do for them. There was no time to sit back and think about what had happened. I had to move forward and we needed to make progress.

When you have a child or children with autism, you meet many different doctors. Some doctors will say or do things that make you not want to continue service with them. I was asked to sign a contract before one doctor would help my child, stating that I would not have any more kids, because I had two kids with autism and there was a chance that any subsequent children might have autism as well. I told him I would not do such a thing. All kids are beautiful, and all kids deserve to live.

We then met a neurologist who was the most amazing woman. She explained everything to me. She was involved with my kids' recovery. She was very informative and resourceful. She gave me hope, and I stayed with her until she retired. She gave me hope because she let me know that with work and commitment, it will get better. She explained to me the therapies that were out there. She told me about amazing people with autism like Mozart, Temple Grandin, and Einstein. That made me feel like my children have a chance to become productive citizens and have amazing lives even with their challenges. My neurologist gave me a diagnosis, but once you get your answer, you cannot stop there. You have to come up with a plan. The kid's neurologist, pediatrician, and psychologist all had input for creating their plan.

Remember to stop and take a deep breath. All of the doctors that care for your child need to be on the same page. This will make everything run smoothly and in order. It will be okay, even if it isn't. Take it one step at a time. Prayer and patience are everything. It's awesome if you have family for support. If you do not have family, create your own supportive circle. I really didn't have family support. It's unfortunate, but what are you going to do? My support became my friends and other parents who also have kids with autism.

I found parents fighting the same fight I am, fighting for recovery. We understand each other and we do not judge each other. It hurts when the people you think will be there aren't. But let that go, and put that energy into what matters—recovery.

Today, my kids have increased their abilities. Their behavior, speech, social skills, and communication have improved. Ryan, my second child, is still a quiet child. He will talk with his favorite cartoons, sing along with his favorite song, play pretend and talk with his favorite toys, and sign for his formula. He was born with a hiatal hernia and reflux. He is not eating solids yet, but he had surgery in December 2013 to treat his reflux and hiatal hernia. I am hopeful he will eat solids soon. His sensory and social skills have improved. He hugs you; he loves to cuddle and sit in groups.

Brian, my first child, is amazing. He is very smart. He is talking and loves to talk, and he's expanding his vocabulary every day. He loves to cook and wants to learn how to make more foods. He is very good at solving problems. His sensory and social skills are skyrocketing. He hugs me, kisses me, and tells me he loves me. I remember the doctor saying I might not ever hear the words "I love you." He was so wrong.

My third child, Zion, is showing signs of autism spectrum disorder (ASD). He is two years old now. I will go through the same steps with him. He is currently in speech and occupational therapy. He improves every day.

I am a parent who's winning with three handsome boys. All three of my boys are gifts from God. I know if I commit and work hard to heal and recover my boys, God will do all the things I cannot do. That's why I will be optimistic. This is faith. God has my family and He has a plan that works beyond my ability. Autism parents are overworked and overwhelmed, but He always comes in to give us that second wind. You need to trust God and walk by faith.

My instruction manual to raise my kids is somewhat different from those of other parents. Parents of kids with autism are judged harshly sometimes because people see our kids only on the surface: "Why is he acting like that?" "Does he cry like that all the time?" "You must not be doing something right." I've heard it all, and I was ripped apart because it mostly came from people who were close to me. Outsiders are quick to say we are bad parents and our children are not disciplined. I would like to say to these people who do not understand: "Do your research. Get to know us. You really do not know the life we live, and we need all the love that someone is willing to give to us."

My journey has taught me compassion, discipline, patience, and the real meaning of love. We are still on the road to recovery, but we have come such a long way. It's a battle. Stick with it.

25

Barracuda
No Guide to Recovery

WHEN I WAS PREGNANT, I READ THE MAYO CLINIC'S *GUIDE TO a Healthy Pregnancy*. I was so excited that I was going to be a mom! It was a rough pregnancy, but Sophia was born healthy, and that was all that mattered to me. She hit all her developmental milestones, but the perfect storm was on the horizon.

It didn't happen overnight; it was a slow regression over six months into what I would come to learn was autism. Between twelve and eighteen months, she had eight ear infections, all treated with antibiotics and lots of Tylenol, plus all of her vaccines. Sound familiar? I had no idea what was happening to Sophia and why she stopped talking. I thought she was sick and that was why she was always crying, had night terrors, screamed all the time, had strange rashes and bad bowel movements, fell down all the time, and wasn't interested in being touched or playing. She had a hearing test and failed, so the doctor recommended tubes. After she had the tubes put in her ears, there was another hearing test and this time she passed.

I thought her words would come back and all the other symptoms would just magically go away.

I enrolled her in an Early Intervention program so she could receive speech therapy. Within a few months, I went from thinking Sophia was catching up and had sensory issues to wondering if there was more to it. Why weren't her words coming back even though she had a speech therapist?

Her sensory issues were getting better, but I started to notice she didn't understand anything I said and was developmentally delayed compared to other two-year-olds. A dear friend told me about a website called Generation Rescue. She said they had a screening test on their website for autism spectrum disorders. I took the screening test, and it indicated autism. It all made sense: the toe walking, staring at ceiling fans, teeth grinding, turning lights on and off, not being able to point or talk. At twenty-five months, the doctor came to our house and assessed Sophia using the Autism Diagnostic Observation Schedule (ADOS). The diagnosis was moderate to severe autism. The doctor went over her recommendations with my husband and me.

The primary recommended therapies were RDI (Relationship Development Intervention, a form of behavioral therapy) and sensory integration by an occupational therapist to address sensory processing disorder. She also suggested we take Sophia to a Defeat Autism Now! (DAN!) doctor named Dr. Berger. It was overwhelming. I thought autism was a disorder that affected boys.

I called Dr. Berger's office the day after my daughter was diagnosed. He had a six-month waitlist. I told my husband we'd have to wait, and I will never forget what came out of his mouth next: "Fuck that! We are starting Sophia on the gluten- and casein-free diet now!"

A few days later, it was Mother's Day. My husband, Eben, gave me two books, *Louder Than Words* by Jenny McCarthy and *The Kid-Friendly ADHD & Autism Cookbook* by Pamela J. Compart, MD, and Dana Laake, RDH, MS, LDN. I read Jenny's book, and Eben read the cookbook.

The first four months after starting Sophia on the gluten- and casein-free diet were like the movie *Groundhog Day*. We'd wake up, have breakfast, Eben would go to work, Sophia would watch *Baby Einstein* (which I know now was visual crack cocaine), the therapists would come to our house, and by mid-morning this weird rash would appear on her face, though it would be gone by the time Eben got home. We observed enough improvements, however, that we stuck with the diet. Sophia was more aware of her surroundings, for instance. Although we saw progress, it was an extremely isolating time for Sophia and me. There were so many challenges, it was hard to go out in public. We had in-home therapy, Eben traveled a ton on business, there was no respite care, and no one wanted to babysit.

In a roundabout way, I found a local chiropractor/nutritionist who had a few patients on the autism spectrum. She recommended an IgG test, and when the results came back, it was an *a-ha!* moment. The test showed she was allergic to eggs, almonds, peanuts, blackberries, raspberries, and garlic. I'd been giving her eggs for breakfast, and all she'd been drinking was almond milk; her favorite fruit was berries. We immediately eliminated those foods and, per the nutritionist's suggestion, started Sophia on a probiotic. During the first week, Sophia had flu-like symptoms and some pretty nasty bowel movements, but the changes were awesome! No more constipation! No more strange rashes and zoning out! No more teeth grinding!

During this time, I got a lot of advice from friends and Sophia's therapists, not all of it welcome. I was so angry at that time that I ended up projecting on many people that were only trying to help. I lost most of my friends, and my isolation was a strain on family, all of whom lived far away and did not understand what it was like to take care of a child that was aggressive, had no sense of danger, had no language, and didn't want to be touched. Back then, the only way I could get eye contact with Sophia was if I roared like a lion.

Fortunately, I met the most dynamic mom. Her name is Kari, and she has two kids on the spectrum. She listened to everything I had to say and very gently guided me to the *Age of Autism* website. Kari and *AoA* became my family. At first she was a mentor to me, but soon she became my best friend. She guided me on the education process, local services and supports, and, most importantly, she listened. I honestly don't know what would have happened if she hadn't entered my life.

At three years of age, Sophia started preschool in the public school system in a blended program. I didn't want Sophia in a contained autism unit, because I didn't want her to be around children that would teach her bad behaviors. She received the maximum amount of therapy in school, and we continued our sprint with behavioral, occupational, horse, and aqua therapies. Having Sophia in school was the first break I'd had in over a year. I no longer felt like I was under house arrest! I met other moms at school and at horse therapy, and I started attending a local support group.

Sophia was doing well with all her therapies, but school was a big disappointment. When I received her progress report at the end of the school year, it was a wake-up call. Sophia wasn't going to make it in a blended class. A mom I'd met at horse therapy advised me to switch to a contained autism unit. She advised me to get all the help I could now, with the goal of going mainstream eventually. It was very hard to admit that I'd been in denial. Sophia had the very same behaviors that I had not wanted her to be exposed to, and a year into diet changes, probiotics, and a few supplements, Sophia was nowhere near recovered.

That summer, Sophia started neurofeedback, a medical therapy that helps improve brain function. First, she had a QEEG (a medical device that displays the electrical brain activity and can identify mental disorders). Sophia's QEEG showed that she had moderate autism. I cried on the way home from the doctor's office, not understanding how she could still be moderate when we'd done all those therapies.

Eben told me not to worry; she'd get better with the neurofeedback therapies called NeuroField and LENS. Practically overnight, Sophia progressed. She started to sometimes point and request with a grunt. It was the beginning of connections. I remember watching *Sesame Street* with Sophia and seeing her laugh at a skit. It brought tears of joy to hear her laugh. RDI had taught us about co-regulation, shared experiences, and joint attention. Easier said than done, but with neurofeedback, it was happening!

The new school year started, and I made the rookie move of telling her new teacher all about neurofeedback. Although there was progress, there were also adverse behaviors from neurofeedback. All of Sophia's negative behaviors at school were then blamed on neurofeedback, and although the progress outweighed the negative, it was hard for Sophia to learn at school. Eben and I met with the doctor and decided to hold off on LENS until Thanksgiving break. It was a really bad time, and the occasional poop smearing that had started when she was two years old turned into a daily event. Eben and I couldn't figure out why this was happening, and, sadly, although she was almost four years old, Sophia was nowhere near ready to be potty trained. Eben and I were fighting a lot over what to do. Although Sophia had made progress, she had now plateaued, and we were losing hope.

I was in a funk, but continued to read *Age of Autism* every day. I especially liked Kim Stagliano, the managing editor of *Age of Autism*, and she mentioned that she had a new book coming out called *All I Can Handle* and would have a book signing party at the National Autism Association conference in St. Pete Beach, Florida. That was only a few miles from where we lived. I asked Eben if we could go, but he said that it wasn't in our budget. Then my brother-in-law came to the rescue and bought us tickets to the conference as an early Christmas gift!

The conference was a game changer. Not only did I meet my hero, Kim Stagliano, but Eben and I also met like-minded parents from all over the country. We saw as many presentations as we could. We drove home talking over each other, so excited and full of hope! Recovery was explained over and over again to be possible. The last day of the conference, Eben attended a presentation on mast cells (cells filled with basophil granules, found in numbers in connective tissue, that release histamine and other substances during inflammatory and allergic reactions) by Dr. Theoharis Theoharides (Dr. Theo), professor of pharmacology, internal medicine, and biochemistry, and the director of Molecular Immunopharmacology and Drug Discovery Laboratory at Tufts University School of Medicine. Afterward, Eben approached me in the lobby and said, "This is it! Hurry! We need to get to their booth!" I couldn't remember the last time I'd seen Eben this excited. As we rushed to the booth, Eben said he could barely keep up during the presentation, which took me aback because he always tracked everything. We got to the booth, which was already crowded, bought a supplement called NeuroProtek that Dr. Theo had formulated, and picked up literature.

I was sad that the conference was over, but Eben and I were back on track. We started Sophia on NeuroProtek, and Eben diligently researched mast cells and brain inflammation. Two weeks later, we left for a much-needed vacation in the Bahamas. I was worried about Sophia's poop smearing, but it wasn't going to stop us. The second day of our trip, I opened Sophia's pull-up and found a perfect bowel movement. I yelled to Eben to get the camera. Yes, I took a picture. This was Sophia's first normal bowel movement since she regressed into autism! We couldn't believe it! Every subsequent day was yet another normal bowel movement. Then Sophia got her first tan. We lived in Florida, and Sophia could be in the sun without sunscreen and she would not get a sunburn or a tan. Neither of us fully understood the critical role of mast cells, but it was obvious NeuroProtek was working. We celebrated Sophia's fourth birthday on our trip. We just knew this was going to be Sophia's break-out year!

Once home, we started back up with neurofeedback. I was nervous, but Eben insisted, and he doesn't take no for an answer, especially when it comes to helping Sophia. Guess what? No side effects! Now, how could that be? Eben tried to explain it to me, but it was way over my head. Finally, he said that NeuroProtek penetrates the blood–brain barrier and reduces inflammation. Okay, but how do I explain this to my friends?

Over the next couple of months, Sophia was on a roll. I hadn't said anything to her teacher. In fact, I didn't even tell her Sophia had resumed neurofeedback. Sophia's eye contact significantly improved. Her teacher was beside herself with excitement. Sophia started to wave! She was trying to be social! She became both sympathetic and empathetic! She was able to use the picture cards at school to communicate! Finally, after a couple of months, her teacher asked me what we were doing, so I came clean. She wanted to understand, so I emailed her some of Dr. Theo's research. Friends, too, noticed the improvements, so I sent them the same information. No one had a clue what all this medical research meant, so I asked Eben to create a document called "Mast Cells for Dummies," which has since morphed into a parent-friendly website on mast cell activation.

Life was really good, but there was one thing I wanted more than anything else in the world. It happened two months after starting NeuroProtek. My first kiss from Sophia! It was magical, and I still get choked up just thinking about it. Her kisses taught me gratitude. I was finally able to move away from all the anger I had in my heart, and it felt wonderful.

The months flew by, and before we knew it, we were in Chicago at our first AutismOne conference. Eben and I had been sharing Sophia's story with Dr. Theo and his team, and it was good to reunite. Sophia had a blast in the child care provided by the Son-Rise Program. Eben primarily hung out at Mast Cell Master booth, and I attended lectures and met the most amazing moms on the planet. Some of those moms went on to create the Thinking Moms'

Revolution. It took us a couple of weeks to come down off our conference high.

That summer, Sophia was doing so well that we could attend a birthday party. She had so much fun swimming and bouncing on the inflatable water slide. Oddly, the next day, Sophia was a different child. I thought she was having seizures, and it scared the shit out of me. I took videos and sent them to her pediatrician, Dr. Berger, Dr. Theo, and her neurologist. Dr. Theo gave me a phone number for another doctor, Martha Herbert, a pediatric neurologist and a brain development researcher, and told me to call her. At the time, I didn't know who she was, but he thought she could help. She not only took my call, but reviewed the videos and asked what we'd done the day before. When I told her about the party she explained that a chlorinated pool can sometimes bring on tics and Tourette's. She then suggested that I contact Boston Children's Hospital, which I did, and they asked me a lot of questions about recent illnesses.

I called my friend Kari and told her I didn't understand why they were asking these questions. Kari asked if there were any other symptoms. I told her about the extreme OCD, frequent urination, major sensory issues, separation anxiety, loud vocalization, and constant stimming. Kari said, "I wonder if it is PANDAS?" (PANDAS is short for Pediatric Autoimmune Neuropsychiatric Disorders Associated with Streptococcal Infections.) *Ding! Ding! Ding!* Thank you, Kari!

I hung up, called the pediatrician, and told him that I thought Sophia had PANDAS. He'd never heard of it, but said to come in the next day. When we arrived, he'd researched PANDAS and did a rapid strep test. The results were negative, but he said that didn't mean anything and wrote a script for azithromycin.

That summer was brutal, and I could write a book on the evils of PANDAS/PANS. Instead, I want to tell you that treating it was a collaborative effort. Thanks to Dr. Berger, Dr. Theo, Dr. Hebert, Scott Smith, Sophia's primary pediatrician, and Dr. Tanya Murphy, Sophia was diagnosed with PANS. I purposely didn't include her neurologist in this list. He ran the ASO test (a blood test to measure antibodies against streptolysin O, a substance produced by group A streptococcus bacterium), an MRI, and twenty-four-hour VEEG, and determined she didn't have PANDAS; he then said she needed to be on an antipsychotic drug. I told him, "The only person that is going to take an antipsychotic is me, so I don't kill you!"

Getting Sophia back took time. The major symptoms were kept at bay with azithromycin and probiotics, but she'd lost all her fine motor skills. She couldn't even use utensils. When she returned to school, her teacher and therapists were shocked. All of Sophia's progress was gone. We had to rewrite her IEP goals. Sophia was on and off azithromycin for ten months. The good news was that after about seven months of having to be held down and forced to swallow pills, she learned how to independently take them! The bad news was that without azithromycin, PANS would always come back.

During my PANS research, I found a website called *Regarding Caroline*. It had an alternative PANDAS protocol. Yes, there was a way to treat PANDAS without antibiotics! So I attended lectures on these alternative protocols at AutismOne to learn more about them. I will never forget meeting Caroline's mom. She empowered me to keep going.

After our first autism conference, Eben began volunteering at conferences, working the Mast Cell Master booth. He has a way of talking to parents and doctors about mast cell activation and the benefits of NeuroProtek. That year, at AutismOne, some of these doctors recommended we try Biocidin in place of azithromycin. Knock on wood—since starting Sophia on Biocidin, she hasn't had a flare! Goodbye, PANS!

Mother's Day always reminds me of Sophia's autism diagnosis. It was 2012, three years after Sophia was diagnosed, and I thought no different from previous years. Eben and I had been working with Sophia on potty training. It didn't take long for Sophia to start urinating on the toilet, but she wasn't able to get to the toilet in time to have a bowel movement. Eben spoke with Dr. Theo, and together they decided to increase Sophia's NeuroProtek dosage. A few days later, Sophia had her first bowel movement on the toilet, on Mother's Day! We opened up a bottle of champagne we'd been saving for a special occasion and celebrated.

Now that Sophia was potty trained, private schools were an option. I found the perfect school that could provide an excellent education and therapies for her. They reviewed her IEP and FBA (behavioral plan) and met her in person, and it looked like she was a good fit. All the school needed was a progress report from her teacher. After they reviewed the report, they determined she would not be able to attend because they couldn't keep her safe. Sophia was a runner, and they weren't equipped to handle runners. I was devastated, but it was for the best in the long run, because Sophia attended a public school that year with an amazing teacher, aides, principal, therapists, and behavior specialist. The school even advocated for a personal aide, and three months into the school year, Ms. B. became Sophia's aide. A few months later, the school got her to stop running!

A mom I'd met at conferences started a weekly Facebook post called FUA (Fuck You Autism). She'd write about something great that her sons had done that week and then asked us to share our stories. At first, I'd post that Sophia didn't do something this week, but it didn't take long for me to catch on. Soon I was on a roll, and everything Sophia did, whether picking her nose or shaking her head to say no, became a FUA accomplishment. It changed the way I thought about Sophia. Celebrating the positives and sharing with other parents is addictive, and to this day, that is what keeps me going.

Time was flying by, and it was conference time again. I'd been looking forward to the National Autism Association conference because the keynote speaker was the one and only Eustacia Cutler.

I'd read her book, *A Thorn in My Pocket*, about raising her daughter, Temple Grandin, and couldn't wait to hear her present. Not only did I hear her and have her sign my book, I even had the privilege of having dinner with Eustacia! She asked me to tell her about Sophia. She didn't like that Sophia was in a contained autism classroom. She went on to tell me about Temple's childhood and the wonderful Montessori school Temple had attended. She said it was there that Temple found her love of animals and learned to play. It sounded wonderful, but I explained that such schools just didn't exist in Florida.

The last day of the conference, I went to the Speech Nutrients booth. I'd tried the Speak supplement when it first came out, but Sophia didn't take pills then and wouldn't drink anything we tried to cut it with, so I gave the bottle away. I completely forgot about it until I heard Dr. Sears's presentation at the conference, in which he mentioned Speak. Duh, she takes pills now! I was going to buy some, but the woman at the booth said, "Why not try it first?" She gave me a month's supply of free samples.

A week into starting Speak, Sophia started to talk! We went to the same park we'd been going to for years, and suddenly she walked over to the rock climbing wall and scaled it! Talk about FUA! Holy guacamole! Sophia had words and gross motor skills! I called the company that makes Speak. I had to understand and explain to, oh, I don't know, everyone that came in contact with Sophia, why suddenly right before her sixth birthday she started talking!

The vice president of the company Speech Nutrients told me that it just wasn't possible. She asked me what else we were doing. I told her we learned the hard way to do only one thing at a time. I then told her that perhaps the NeuroProtek we'd used for the past two years optimized the results of Speak. Who really knows why, but it worked. Sophia went from preverbal to verbal in a week. Did she instantly start talking like her peers? Hell no, but who really cares? She went from hurting me every day to saying, "No." The word "no" was music to my ears. Even now, a year into Sophia talking, hearing her say "Mommy" just melts my heart.

In the meantime, I heard a rumor that our local Montessori school was starting an autism program. Could it be true? I called the school and scheduled a meeting. Yes, it was true, and they asked if I could share my resources on autism and sensory processing disorder along with the best therapists and teachers in the area. They asked me what my wish list was for this pilot program and said yes to everything, except converting their pool to a saltwater system. I cried—not because of the pool, but because they not only listened to me, but they said yes, and the pilot program was formed and in place within the year.

Sophia is now at that school and thriving! Ironically, the name of Sophia's school is the same as that of Temple Grandin's childhood school. To be honest, I never thought that Sophia would come this far in school. She is learning cursive and multiplication, has no need for an FBA, and is reading! I post every gain on Facebook because it gives me strength, and I believe Sophia is a better person. FUA! Never give up!

Update

Two years have passed since I wrote this chapter. We no longer live in Florida, but before we moved out of state last summer, Sophia continued her journey on recovery road with so many FUA milestones I lost count. In the spring of 2014, Sophia started Brain Balance, a program that addresses academic, social, and behavioral issues. Our family felt that she could benefit from hemispheric integration therapies offered at Brain Balance, but everything is so expensive! My in-laws came to the rescue.

Two weeks into Brain Balance, Sophia said her first sentence to me, which was clear as day: "Can I have a pedicure, please?" Thank goodness she didn't ask for a horse. Then her second sentence came a few days later. At the health food store, the butcher asked her what she wanted, and she replied, "Can I have the ribeye steak, please?" I looked down at the price—it was $16.99 per pound for organic grass-fed steak. I asked for the smallest one, and my husband and I ate chicken that night.

She was a happy child but with ups and downs, and we just kind of went into cruise mode. Then I got sick. We moved to Massachusetts in Fall 2015. It was time to stop with my continued health decline and be near family and live in a place that could support my immune system. Sophia has continued progressing; she is in a wonderful public school that has an amazing special education program and—wait for it—yep, true inclusion with time in a mainstream classroom! She has friends and is thriving!

At the beginning of every year, my husband and I put together and try to prioritize a New Year's resolution for Sophia's recovery road. This year, we really wanted to try a specific footbath from a company called AMD (A Major Difference). Unfortunately, we had recently bought a house, so the AMD purchase wasn't in our budget. So I called AMD and asked if there were any local practitioners in my area that offered this footbath therapy.

I was in luck—the person I spoke with was very kind and gave me the name and phone number of someone near us. We started the therapy, and saw enough gains that we decided that when we got our tax return, we would invest in this.

Before that could happen, we experienced an unexpected game changer. FedEx arrived at our house six weeks ago with a big box. When I opened it, I saw a huge red bow with a tag that read "Sophia, I adore you. You inspire me every day! Love, C."

I knew what it was and became a hot mess. I called my husband, and we made a plan. He would leave work early and I'd pick Sophia up from school; then we'd meet up at our house, get our phones ready, and take pictures as we watched her open what she had wanted since September—the AMD footbath she tried last fall at Autism Education Summit. It was a very exciting day.

We believe Sophia is going to make it! I don't care about the autism. I care about the subset of illnesses that often are disregarded with the casual comment: "Oh, don't worry—that is just autism." No fucking way! I don't buy that one bit! FUA! Never ever give up!

26

Rebel
God Doesn't Make Junk

My story begins June 16, 1998. My family and I had recently returned home in April after living as expats for three and a half years in the United Kingdom. It was time to take my two-year-old daughter to her well-child visit. As a mom who was seriously interested in the best health care for her children, I dutifully brought my daughter to a pediatrician in Germantown, Maryland, whom I had carefully interviewed beforehand. At the time, I had no reason to mistrust doctors.

The only odd thing I remember about this appointment is that I had to sign a form prior to my daughter being given her annual vaccines. I remember asking the nurse why I had to sign my name before the DTaP and the Hib were administered. She said, "Oh, it is something we do now." In hindsight, this should have been a red flag. You generally do not sign for something unless there is a reason. Liability comes to mind. Of course, all I was given was the normal instructions: "If she runs a fever, give her Tylenol." They say this to you very nonchalantly, like it is perfectly commonplace.

In the evening, my daughter ran a very high fever. I heard her crying and, in my middle-of-the-night stupor, took her to bed with me. I did not take her temperature, but I was shocked at how hot she felt. I dutifully gave her Tylenol, which, I found out later, gave her body less ability to fight the toxic insults of the vaccine. Her fever came down, and I thought no more of it. I found out several years later that Tylenol lowers glutathione levels. (Glutathione is our body's major antioxidant, detoxifier, and regulator of ATP.) The effects of her vaccine-induced brain injury began appearing very soon.

It was customary for my family to attend the fireworks display each Independence Day, and this year was no different. I noted that this time, instead of enjoying the excitement of the fireworks, my toddler screamed the entire time. As a young mother, I thought this was odd. My daughter had attended fireworks displays before and had never had a problem with them.

As time went on, my daughter became known in the family as our love bug. She always wanted hugs and, of course, we all obliged her. She wanted hugs because her body craved deep pressure. My daughter did not feel grounded. She also was petrified of elevators and escalators, a fear that at times became a real inconvenience. How do you shop in a fancy mall while avoiding elevators and escalators? I can also recall when we were at West Point burying my father-in-law, and my daughter again refused to go in the elevator. At the time, I thought, *Why is my child so out of sync? Why is her behavior so difficult?* The grandparents looked at this behavior and blamed me for the behavioral oddities they saw. "You are not disciplining her enough," I often heard.

Eventually, other problems began appearing. Around the age of five, my daughter was doing a writing exercise with her cousin, who was a year behind her, under the instruction of her grandmother, who had a background in special education. My mother-in-law noticed that my daughter was behind in her fine motor skills—she could not keep up with her cousin in this writing exercise. My mother-in-law mentioned her concern to me that day, but I brushed it off. Who wants to think about their child being behind?

We never discussed specifics, but I know now my daughter was struggling with holding a pencil properly. Years later we would have an occupational therapist come to the house to help with this.

I was still very much in the dark about what had happened to my daughter, so she continued receiving the required vaccines.

I began to take note of other developmental delays. When my daughter reached second grade, she was still struggling to tie her shoes and ride her bike. She also still wanted to be carried. I did not know it at the time, but my daughter had trouble moving through space. It was also very difficult to transition her to different activities. Eating as a family was almost impossible. My daughter's brain could not unfocus from what she was paying attention to at the time. When she did finally come to the table, her food would still be too hot, and she would still have to wait until she could tolerate the food temperature.

School was also becoming a nightmare. My daughter was begging me to homeschool her. I think it was because her environment at school was very negative. At the time I did not know she had a vision processing disorder, sensory processing disorder, and an auditory processing disorder. Her eyes could not track or focus, which affected her comprehension. She also was not able to hear her teacher if there was any background noise.

The complaints were coming in from her teachers, as well—lack of focus during instruction and seatwork time, hard time staying on task, spending too much time visiting with her classmates at her table, difficulty listening and following directions, not putting in her best effort, and being unable to manage her time. It was common for a short period of time for schools to perform a Connor's Rating Scale for students who were inattentive to instruction. When my daughter was assessed, she scored in the 99th percentile on the ADHD index!

I will never forget the next doctor's visit. I armed myself with her schoolwork and records to ensure that the pediatrician could get a clear understanding of the cognitive difficulties my daughter was encountering in school. The doctor never looked at them. She spent very little time with us; she just handed us a psychotropic drug, Strattera, and sent us on our way. A pill for every ill, right? I left feeling very disillusioned, but I went along with it. After all, trust your doctor, right? Maybe a pill *would* fix all of this? It seemed like she might have experienced some improvement in school for the next six months, but it might have been due to her transferring to a charter school with a laid-back teacher. Whatever the cause, the improvements stopped after six months. Moreover, the medication had also affected her appetite and caused my daughter to lose weight she did not need to lose.

From there, it was drugs, drugs, and more drugs. Drugs were prescribed for her ADHD and for her problems with sleeping. If one drug did not work, we would be given another one to try. Her sleep study revealed she never reached REM sleep.

This is how a typical morning went in my house: I would literally have to drag my daughter out of bed. She would get dressed as long as it was not cold in her room. If it was cold, she would not leave her bed. When she made her way downstairs, she would lie down on the couch and sleep. The drug given to help with her sleep clearly was not working. (It would be later confirmed through genetic testing that my daughter had a mitochondrial disorder. The mitochondria regulate the energy of the cell.)

My daughter's breakfast consisted of a breakfast bar or dry cereal on the way to school (if she was not sleeping). Once we got to school, it was another fight to get her out of the car. I remember how the drugs would cause her to talk nonstop. This was very scary to watch. I also remember looking at her dilated pupils. Now, in hindsight I ask myself, "What are we doing to these kids?"

She continued to fall behind in school. Math tutoring began in fourth grade. Passing the FCAT, a required state test in Florida, had eluded her since third grade. Her fifth grade teacher told me they had to rub her back to keep her on task. I tried several times over the years to get her an Individualized Educational Plan, but I was unsuccessful. The IEP is important for helping your child to learn how she learns and to test how she tests. For example, she should always have a reader when she tests. She also should have unlimited testing time. I was told that because she was a "B" student, she did not qualify for an IEP. She was too smart. Her doctor wrote a letter indicating that my daughter should never be given timed tests. The letter was ignored by the school because the principal did not believe in ADHD.

She did her best in school in fifth grade, when she was chosen to perform in *Miracle on 34th Street* with the Orlando Repertory Company. This involved performing four shows a week during school and on weekends for six weeks. The school principal was very much against this because she did not want my daughter to miss that much school. In fact, she requested that I disenroll her and never bring her back. I had to get the school attorney involved because what the principal was telling me to do was illegal. I marvel now at how we were able to pull this off despite all my daughter was going through.

As all this was happening, I was looking for answers about what might be wrong. There have been many *a-ha!* moments on this journey. On the last day of fifth grade, I heard these words from her teacher, "Your daughter is not in the classroom." I made a decision right then and there that I would have her cognitively tested before she entered sixth grade, and that she would have an IEP in place prior to starting middle school.

The summer before sixth grade, we began what is called a neuropsychological exam. My daughter was not the most cooperative and sometimes she would refuse to test. At times, Dr. H. could not get her to focus on testing. We finished the testing with help from a female intern—changing something or making the circumstances different can sometimes lead to cooperation with children on the autism spectrum.

During this time, my oldest daughter was also working with a neuropsychologist because she had received a diagnosis of ADD the summer of her junior year of high school. It turned out that this neuropsychologist, Dr. G., actually trained Dr. H. After Dr. H. completed the testing, he gave my daughter the diagnoses of Oppositional Defiant Disorder, depression, and ADHD.

One of the recommendations on the report included the Interactive Metronome, a program my older daughter was doing for her ADD at the time. This program involves movements that cross the mid-line of the body with hands and feet to the beat of the metronome. So my next stop was back to Dr. G. to see if the Interactive Metronome would be an appropriate therapy for my youngest daughter. I was sitting in Dr. G.'s office, having handed him the neuropsychological results. He walked out of his office with the report in his hand, shaking his head, and told me the diagnosis from Dr. H. was not right. He said my daughter had autism. He made sure to specify that she did not have Asperger's; instead, it was Pervasive Developmental Disorder-Not Otherwise Specified. Given my limited knowledge of autism back then, all I knew was that it was not a positive diagnosis.

Not wanting to lose any hope, I asked him if Interactive Metronome Therapy could still help my daughter. The look on his face said it all. I could try, he said. I got the feeling that he had no hope for my daughter. The whole time my daughter was lying on my lap appearing completely out of it. Dr. G. gave us referrals for life skills, social skills, and for a vision processing specialist. I left the office stunned but determined to beat this autism, as well as find out what it really was, what caused it, and how it happened. My life as an independent researcher and an avid reader began.

Our next appointment involved an evaluation by an occupational therapist. At this appointment, I learned more. My daughter had low muscle tone and muscle strength. She also had significant deficits in bilateral integration, upper limb coordination, and balance skills, as well as auditory, proprioceptive, and vestibular deficits. Finally some of her problems were starting to make sense: holding her pencil with her fist, her difficulty in riding a bike, her fear of riding escalators and elevators, why she never runs, and why she could not hear me if there was any background noise.

It came time for my daughter's IEP meeting. I was prepared. I came in with a child advocate, my husband, my daughter's picture, my daughter's school reports going all the way back to kindergarten, and most importantly, information stating the law from wrightslaw.com. My daughters PDD-NOS diagnosis fell under the category of "other health impaired," which includes limited alertness with respect to the educational environment. Obtaining the services of a child advocate who is not a lawyer to represent you is advised because of the emotions involved. (Who represents you varies from state to state as does the process. Some states require you obtain a lawyer.)

When you enter these meetings, you will find yourself outnumbered. I think this is done on purpose to intimidate the parents—after all, money is involved. The school loses money if you decide your child would benefit from leaving the public school system. Once an Individualized Educational Plan is granted, your child becomes eligible for a McKay Scholarship in our state. This scholarship allows for attendance in an approved private school. This was my end game. Fortunately, I had a good relationship with the school counselor because he knew my middle daughter, who was in the gifted program. He knew I am an educated parent whose demands were very reasonable given the circumstances. At one point in the meeting, it looked like they were leaning toward putting my daughter in a school where kids who struggle cognitively are separated from the neurotypical kids and the academic require-ments are dumbed down.

I was prepared, however, and I quoted the law I described above. The whole mood changed. I heard the words "other health impair-ment" and I knew I had won.

My daughter was now eligible for the McKay Scholarship! We chose a Montessori School, because I liked how the students were allowed to work at their own pace. I also knew the owner and felt my daughter would be taught in a way that she learns and tests. One advantage is the classes are much smaller. Teachers in private schools also see more of these kids who struggle cognitively and have more knowledge about how to get them to perform in a positive way.

While we were there, the school screened for speech and lan-guage skills. My daughter's screening indicated she had language deficits and needed further testing. We followed through and paid out of pocket to find out she had language deficits that mimicked a traumatic brain injury. She had never had a traumatic brain injury, unless you count the damage that was done by the vaccines.

For the next two years, my daughter would attend three more schools. We left the Montesorri school the next year because Maria was struggling in Math, and her teacher, who was a family member of the principal, struggled with this subject too, and I knew he would never be asked to leave his position. We left the next school because my daughter would have been the only girl in the class if she stayed. The next school we left because my daughter really wanted to go back to the public school and be involved in the show choir, like her sisters were.

Sometimes new problems would appear. It was during puberty that violence came into play. You never knew when she would have a meltdown out of nowhere, with another one soon to follow. A melt-down consisted of finding the nearest object regardless how heavy it was and heaving it in my direction. I found myself in a constant state of post-traumatic stress disorder. Thankfully, she was able to hold it together in school.

While my daughter was in middle school, a hair analysis test for heavy metal toxicity was given to me by a doctor we were seeing from the College of Vision Development. The results of this test gave me my next *a-ha*! moment.

The testing results revealed my daughter was off the charts in copper, magnesium, and very high in manganese. My holistic pediatrician referred me to a DAN! doctor, whom he was shadowing at the time. I was told by the DAN! doctor to detoxify her slowly with Epsom salt baths every day for one week. He also prescribed liposomal glutathione to begin the following week. Within days of the start of the Epsom salt baths, I knew we were on our way to healing because of the calming effect I was witnessing. I am particularly proud of an accomplishment involving this doctor. It is unusual to have insurance cover the less-traditional treatments, and I was the first mom in his practice to win my insurance case with Aetna and receive full coverage of care! Becoming a researcher extraordinaire paid off. As an independent researcher, I spent numerous hours on the computer matching my daughter's symptoms with the research that was on pubmed.gov. (This is like the Library of Congress, except it is medical.)

Detox was just the beginning of her journey to recovery, and many problems linger. Chronic fatigue to this day remains a constant symptom in my daughter's life. In high school it became so debilitating that at one point my daughter would come home from high school and sleep for five hours. Because I was an original member of the Autism-Mitochondrial task force, based in Boston, mitochondrial disorder was also on my radar. I frequently had the opportunity to hear specialists and other mothers talk about symptoms I have also observed in my daughter.

In July 2011, I made the decision to buy a water ionizer that produces living alkaline water for my daughter. The scientific name for this water is electrolyzed reduced water. This water is the thinnest water on the planet. It is able to increase oxygen and blood flow in the body. This water is also very high in antioxidants, a quality that can be measured by an ORP (Oxidation Reduction Potential) meter. It is also important that the ionizer has a filtration system that can produce water in its purest form.

When my daughter began drinking living water, she went from sleeping five hours after school to one hour, and she had her best school-year attendance ever! Unfortunately, this came to an end the following year because her classroom teachers discouraged the students from using bathroom passes and offered extra credit instead, which my daughter sorely needed, so she stopped drinking the water. When you drink the thinnest water on the planet, you have to go when nature calls!

Where are we in our journey to wellness these days? I feel like we are still climbing the hill. My daughter recently agreed to visit a holistic doctor who uses electrodermal screening by measuring the frequencies in the organs. The doctor then matches her findings up with over 500 different kinds of remedies. I found out what "autism" means when it comes to my daughter's body. Autism, in my daughter, is mercury, toxoplasmosis, H. pylori, parasites, compromised liver, leaky gut, and hypoglycemia. The word *autism* does not even come close to describing the gravity of how compromised these children are both physically and cognitively.

We came home with an overwhelming array of supplements, tinctures, and a soak. Following this protocol lasted two weeks, and then my daughter refused to take any more. It did not help that my husband thought this was hocus pocus and had openly stated so in front of my daughter.

In the last few months my daughter has embraced the gluten-, casein-, dairy-, and sugar-free diet. Currently, at age seventeen, she still suffers from severe anxiety, so she can no longer attend school while it is in session, and going to the movies is currently a challenge for her. Chronic fatigue is still present. She is starting to become open to taking supplements again and she recognizes she has health challenges that are holding her back. She is now willing to explore this further. My daughter is currently seeing a licensed clinical social worker at my husband's insistence for her anxiety and depression.

When I look at the positive side, I turn to the fact that my daughter is very talented in singing. Her strength lies in the right side of her brain, where she is extremely high functioning. Most days you will find her rehearsing for her next leading role and taking online classes. My daughter has perfect pitch, plays the piano by ear, has a passion for musical theater, and a keen eye for photography.

Update

I penned this chapter when my daughter was seventeen. She has now turned twenty. With a lot of help from her dad, she was able to graduate from high school two months late at a county-wide summer graduation. She missed graduating with her class because of her health issues. After graduation, she worked for a year in a theme park. However, she found herself struggling with her voice because her job involved talking over crowds of people. Because she is a singer, her voice is very important to her. She tried to get into the entertainment part of the company, but so far this has eluded her.

After one year of employment, she turned in her resignation. After three months of looking for work, she is now working in retail and will soon be working at Universal as a photographer. She has also obtained her learner's permit and is currently taking biweekly driving lessons. We found an instructor who is aware of the challenges that kids on the autism spectrum face in regard to the processing and spatial orientation needed when you learn to drive.

She also continues to take voice lessons and attends auditions as opportunities come up. Last summer she took on the role of Laurey in the musical *Oklahoma*, and in May she will be debuting at our local Fringe Festival in a play called *Snappy's Happy Half Hour*.

My daughter is coming to the realization that if she wants to live with her sister in NYC, she needs to start learning how she can support her body so she can experience a normal state of wellness.

We recently learned through genetic testing by MEDomics that she has known mutations in her genes currently implicated in mitochondrial disease or autism spectrum disorder. These are OPA1, SYNE1, and TSC2. This proves my daughter should have never been vaccinated because these mutations indicate that her body is not able to detoxify the heavy metals that are present in the vaccines.

Genetic testing should be a prerequisite before any vaccination to test for any risk factors. No one person is genetically the same, and, therefore, the same vaccine and drug protocol should not be practiced on everyone. It is time for mainstream medicine to start treating everyone as an individual.

I will leave you thinking about what I believe today is the truth about vaccines. Vaccines inflame our brains, delete our DNA, cause microflora dysfunction, lower our immune system, reduce oxygen and blood flow, and compromise our primary reflexes that relate to the functioning of the left and right side of our body and brain. I cannot help but believe that "autism" is intentional. I believe it is intentional because we now have a whistleblower at the Centers for Disease Control who has admitted to committing fraud in regard to the findings in children who received the MMR vaccine prior to age three. The real data was hidden and tampered with, causing harm to hundreds of children.

"Autism" does not reflect the greatness that our Creator intended for us to be. Psalm 139 says, "I praise you because I am fearfully and wonderfully made; your works are wonderful, I know that full well." I will not stop recovering my daughter until she reaches that greatness that God intended not only for her, but for us all.

As this chapter goes to print my daughter has just left to live with her older sister in NYC and pursue her dream to be on Broadway!

27

Muscle Mama
From Denial to Fighting

"IT SHOULDN'T BE THIS HARD." THIS IS WHAT MY HUSBAND SAID to me as he stood in our kitchen in our third home in Missouri, watching me as I wrestled our sixteen-month-old down to the ground, trying to put his shoes on just so we could go outside. Hard? This wasn't hard . . . training thirty-six hours a week as a national gymnast at age sixteen while going to school full-time was hard . . . dieting for five years and competing nationally as a fitness competitor while holding down two jobs was hard . . . moving to the United States as a Canadian, a newlywed, and having to leave behind my career, family and friends, and everything familiar to me was hard. This was just my son being stubborn, as he always was, day in day out, and it just meant I wasn't working hard enough with him.

"I raised my nephew, and I know how a child this age should act. It shouldn't be this difficult," my husband continued to say, after I had finally succeeded in getting our son's shoes on, his little face wet with tears. "He's fine, and it'll get easier," I told him. Surprise, surprise, it never did.

Then, one day, my husband threw the word "autism" at me. My heart almost stopped beating. What? Autism? How could our son have autism? I spent all day, every day, with this kid, so I would be the one to know if something was wrong. Nope, no way. I just needed to try harder. Talk about denial at its best.

My husband saw what I did not. A few weeks later, he came home with some literature explaining what autism is along with some descriptions of case studies. Apparently, he had been speaking to a co-worker who also had a son on the autism spectrum, and my husband was convinced that our precious little boy was headed down that same road. His co-worker had suggested we get an appointment with a neurologist as soon as possible just to make sure, so that if our son did have autism, then at least he would have a medical diagnosis that would allow him to receive services.

At this point, I was angry. I took my husband's actions very personally and as a full assault on my mothering skills, so in protest I threw the information he brought home into the garbage. I responded with: "I think you're wrong, and I'm going to prove it." I was so convinced that I was right that I called the local school district to set up an appointment for preschool screening, and then the neurologist to set up an appointment to confirm my beliefs. How dare my husband think our child had issues when, according to our current pediatrician, he was meeting all of his developmental milestones? He might be difficult, but he sure as hell did not have autism.

A few weeks later, a nice woman from our local school district showed up at our door with toys in hand and forms for me to fill out while she tested Kameron on our living room floor. By the time she was done, she had grown very quiet and then gently showed me the results. She said he had scored in the black, and I remember asking her what that meant. "It's usually an indicator that he needs further testing." *Oh great, what does that mean?* Suddenly, a sinking feeling came over me, and I asked her flat out if she thought he had autism. She replied that she was not qualified enough to make that kind of decision, but she highly recommended we get further testing.

It was early spring, and one of our neighbors decided to host a "social tea" with some other gals in the neighborhood, giving me an opportunity to meet some new people. I became quick friends with a fellow mom who also had a son close to Kameron's age. As we discussed our boys, I of course told her about my recent event with the early childhood center and their findings. She quickly recommended her developmental pediatrician and suggested that I go see her right away. So I called and scheduled a meet and greet with her doctor, whom I will refer to as "Dr. M." I wasn't sure how Dr. M. would tell me anything different from what our former pediatrician had said, but my son's early childhood test results were still haunting me, and I wanted to be sure.

She was very friendly and kind, and waited patiently as I went down my list of concerns and disappointments about prior visits to other pediatricians about the same issues. Oddly enough, Kameron had remained calm throughout this visit—any other time we stepped foot into a doctor's office, he would scream inconsolably until we left. So I looked over at him and noticed he was using my velvet hair scrunchie, which was his comfort object that we never left the house without, and was rubbing it up and down his arms. I thought this was kind of strange, but was happy that he was actually being quiet enough that I could have my conversation with the doctor. When I was done, she looked at me and said, "Has anyone ever mentioned the word autism to you?" I told her not yet, but my husband had had some suspicions. She told me that both what I had explained to her and what she was observing pointed to autism and sensory integration issues.

She suggested we look into the First Steps program, a service provided by the state for kids with special needs, and that we needed to get him in right away. In that moment, my heart sank, the room got smaller, and I started to cry. Dr. M. looked at me; I think she felt horrible that this was this first time I was hearing this. She handed me a tissue and tried to console me, but our time was up because this had only been a meet and greet appointment. Had she known, she would have booked us more time. I told her that it was okay, that I would go. I thanked her for her advice, took my information, and left to go home. I fought so hard to hold back the tears as I left the building, and how I even drove home is still a blur to me.

So this was real . . . not only was there something wrong with my son, but it also had a name and it was what I had feared most. Autism. I had no idea what it was or what it meant for him. My husband had been right and I had been wrong. As soon as we got home, I broke the news to him, and it only verified his suspicions. "Let's wait and see what the neurologist says, and then we'll know for sure." Our appointment was still three weeks away, so now what? Well, for the next three weeks I cried daily, wondering how this happened to us, to our son. How did he get this? And it had a name. A horrible, ugly "A" name that I couldn't even bring myself to say for the longest time because it made me so angry to say it. I even referred to it as the "A-word" for the longest time, and it was never spoken by me in our home.

So all the difficulty that I had with him, which started at around thirteen months of age, had been one of the biggest signs of autism. Regression. We didn't have a clue that it was even happening (though we felt something wasn't right) because it manifested itself slowly enough that an untrained eye wouldn't have noticed right away. By sixteen months, he had lost all his speech and pointing skills, and then the aggression started. When he didn't get what he wanted, he would resort to eye gouging, hair pulling, and even scratching and biting. I used to wonder how this little person could be so angry all the time? How naive had I been?

A good way to describe regression is to say it's like watching your child die right in front of you, but yet they are still there, walking around and breathing. No matter how hard you try you to reach them, you can't. Nothing you do helps, so you stand back and watch helplessly as your child becomes worse and withdraws more into himself every day. Not being able to help your child is one of the worst feelings in the world. You wonder if you will ever feel different.

I think the toughest part for me as a mother during this time was that I knew that my child needed me, relied on me, and depended on me, but there was no connection or acknowledgment of any kind. This expressionless little round face would just stare blankly back, and it was never directly at me, just slightly somewhere past me. There were no sweet sounds, no smiles; no intimate snuggling that a mother and child share. Just a rigid child who screamed when he didn't get what he wanted because he had no words; he screamed himself to sleep because self-soothing could not be learned. He woke up every night and stayed awake for three hours at a time because his sensory issues would completely override his nervous system. Every day he led me around the house by my finger hoping I could figure out what he wanted.

It was finally time for our neurologist appointment. We saw a doctor, whom I will refer to as "Dr. C." He was much younger than I had expected, and his short time in his profession was reflected in his bedside manner—he had horrible sympathy skills. He asked us a lot of questions while observing Kameron, who was well across the other side of the room, sitting comfortably in his stroller, and, again rubbing my velvet scrunchie all along his arms. Then we moved onto the physical part of the examination, and, of course, Kameron started to scream because we had removed him from his safe place in his stroller. Once the doctor had completed his exam, he sat back behind his desk, looked us straight in the eyes, and said: "Your son has autism. You can call it Asperger's or whatever else you want, but it is autism." He then pulled out a handout with a case study about a boy with autism, and then the appointment was over.

He didn't say "Good luck" or "I'm sorry, I know this is a lot to take in right now," just "Here's an explanation of what your child has, and we are done." I was speechless as we walked back to our car, and that horrible sinking feeling consumed me again. This time, my husband was the one to take the brunt of the devastation, the help-lessness, and then the despair, because his worst fear had just been confirmed. His world came crashing down around him. He spent the rest of the day at home with us instead of going back to work, with a bottle of whisky that he nursed in a glass all day. I remember looking out at him through the window, while he stood motionless outside, watching Kameron attempt to play in our backyard, and I could see all of his dreams for Kameron slowly fall from his heart, one by one, and crash to the ground. It's a moment I will never forget. All the dreams that every father has for their firstborn son died that day.

We found solace in each other's arms later that night, holding onto each other tightly, wondering what was to come. We had so many questions with no answers. How were things going to be for us? For him? And for the new baby inside of me that was now at eleven weeks of gestation? How were we going to do this? How was I going to do this alone while my husband worked all day? Where would my support system be when all of my family lived in Canada? Who was going to help me?

As the next few months unfolded, we were thrown into meet-ings, and testing, and pages of paperwork to fill out, and then more testing, and therapists, and it seemed to go on and on. Because Kameron was two years and four months old at his diagnosis, we had a lot to get done before he turned three; otherwise he would be too old to qualify for the First Steps program. So we got to work. We tested him for placement at our local school for their early childhood program, we set up our in-home ABA program, and then managed to qualify to get into the Judevine Center for Autism for a three-week boot camp for families with kids on the spectrum. I was now very pregnant with our daughter trying to juggle all of this, and an emotional hot mess trying to grasp all of the change going on around us. I was extremely overwhelmed by the intensity and speed at which things had to be done.

Finally, one of the therapists scheduled to work with us took pity on me and told me there was a mom that I just had to meet. She had a little boy Kameron's age and was going through the same thing; they were just a little further ahead in their journey. This is when I met "M," to whom I commonly referred later as my angel. She became my saving grace, the support system I so desperately needed. She would become the one to help me navigate through a world that was so uncertain and turbulent, and to find strength and courage in my most desperate times. She was the one I cried with and shared my anger with, as well as my triumphs (they were small, and few and far between, but triumphs nonetheless).

We talked about IEPs and ABA therapists, biomedical doctors, the latest therapies that were slowly surfacing in the autism world, and sometimes even about each other, when the rare opportunity presented itself. Our families became friends, and it was so nice to finally spend time with someone who didn't need an explanation of why our child was doing what he was doing. It was just understood.

We finally began to experience and embrace our "new family dynamic." It wasn't what the normal families of America were experiencing, but it was definitely a step up from where we had started. And it was going to be okay.

I look back on those years, and I am amazed at how I got through those very dark times. I slipped into a deep depression, was extremely sleep deprived, and put on a lot of weight. Even though I had "M" to fall back on, I still became so immersed into my son's world that I sometimes forgot what it was like to function in a world without autism. Thank goodness we had our daughter, because she would quickly snap me out of it and remind me that there was another little person who needed my attention, love, and compassion. She would, as the years went by, become my ticket to a world I thought I would never be a part of again, one that in earlier years I had resented so much. The best part was that every smile, every hug, and every giggle that came out of her was for me and me alone, and slowly our family dynamic changed. Not only because she demanded it, but also because Kameron's journey was changing direction. We were all in this together, as difficult as some of those times were, and she was determined to be a part of everything; from therapy sessions to playdates to daily interactions, she always saw him as her brother and never treated him as having a disability. Her strength and determination to interact with him always her first priority, and she never gave up on him, even if he didn't want to play with her or walked in the other direction. She got in his face when needed and eventually he would come around, even if it was only for a little while. She took and reveled in every moment she could.

The next few years revolved around therapists in our home almost every day, sometimes twice a day for ABA, RDI (Relationship Development Intervention therapy), listening therapy (which is special frequency and pitched type of music that helps stimulate the brain in different ways), and private speech sessions. We transformed our basement into an amazing sensory gym because Kameron suffered from sensory integration issues on a very high level, and, if not regulated properly, these can lead to attention and focus issues, hyperactivity, and sometimes even aggression or injury-inflicting behavior. Our sensory gym became the new home to our continuing ABA program. This basement was so awesome that we hosted both our children's birthday parties in it numerous times. It included everything from an indoor rotational therapy swing to a huge ball pit, which was just an empty inflatable pool filled with balls; a roller machine, aka a squeezing machine, in which Kameron would insert himself into the middle of two rollers that delivered deep, squeezing pressure on both sides; and a bouncy house. My daughter soon became the girl with the "cool basement," and slowly she started to realize some of the perks that came with having a sibling with autism.

Another move transpired, but this time it was back to Michigan, which I dreaded and resisted on every level. After being in Missouri and having access to so many wonderful resources, I knew I was in for a huge disappointment, especially after visiting the schools in the areas we were looking to move into. But in light of my disappointment, this is when I met TMR's SNAP! even before she had become SNAP!. She introduced me to HBOT (hyperbaric oxygen therapy) and many other amazing interventions; she became my new angel. We bonded quickly and banded together to conquer the school system and autism as we knew it. We spent many afternoons discussing our anger and frustrations with a school system that seemed so broken. We had to fight for every single tiny inch of services that we knew our children needed but that they deemed unnecessary or unable to provide due to "staffing issues." We were determined to fix that and fight hard no matter what it took. SNAP! kept me focused and kept me strong, and in the process we became dear friends.

Our struggles played a dominant force on our journey with what I prayed would be recovery; for example, Kameron was not successfully potty trained until six years of age. He did not want to venture into dark places ever, especially barns, making school trips to a farm very difficult. Hearing his sister cry was the biggest challenge, because he would physically go after her to shut her up, and if I didn't get there in time to intervene, he'd usually try to rip her hair out, or scratch her face, or squeeze her arms so tight it left marks. Having to police my children every hour was no easy task, but it was just one more thing that just needed to be done.

The biggest demon and challenge for us: transitions. Getting my son to start anything that wasn't initiated by him or getting him to leave something that he was heavily engrossed in were activities so difficult I felt like a prisoner in my own home. Leaving the house was difficult, getting dressed to go outside was difficult, going to the doctor or the store was difficult, going to the park was especially difficult. The only way to accomplish any of these things was by bringing certain comfort items wherever he went; as he got older, having a written schedule for almost every part of his day became a necessity and a blessing.

Thank goodness he was diagnosed with hyperlexia (a strong affinity for letters and numbers) at a very young age by a speech pathologist who was part of our initial testing in the early years. When she told us he was able to sight read, a door had finally opened for us. The specialist told us to label everything in our home that he came into contact every day. With a lot of tough love, we would make him read the labels, and he wouldn't get what he wanted until he pointed to it—in the earlier days; later on, as his speech progressed, he had to say it as well. Being able to visually see the words attached to each item was soothing and enlightening to him, and finally the world surrounding him started to make sense. As he got older, if he was mad or frustrated with what was going on around him, he learned to ask me to "write it down." This meant he needed me to write down his new schedule because he wanted to make sure no more changes would be made, and at some point there was a beginning to the end of this new schedule. Once those words were on that page and they were numbered in a sequential order, life was good and he was able to move on.

So where are we now? Well, we ended up moving one more time and now live in a small town in the state of Illinois. Kameron just turned thirteen years old. This birthday came with a lot of emotions for me. First, I had a lot of disbelief that I now officially have a teenager. Second, I had a lot of sadness because I had made up my mind, many years ago on our journey, that I was determined to have him recovered by the time he turned thirteen. Unfortunately, that day has not yet come for us, and we are still fighting the big fight.

Is he better? Yes. Has he made progress? Absolutely! This young man went from being a non-verbal, aggressive, and severely autistic little boy to a teenager who now looks me in the eyes and smiles. He now can deliver two to three exchanges in a conversation, will seek me out when he has a comment or a question (which does not come easy to him), and, most importantly, can tell me that he loves me. It took him nine years to do that independently, but he did it, and with such tenderness that, for me, it was one of our biggest victories.

He will engage with his sister occasionally, but he always shares a deep concern for her, especially regarding her emotions and mood, as any older brother would. He loves to hear her sing, and he has quite the singing voice himself. We discovered just recently by total coincidence that he is extremely talented on the piano, and he will now be participating in the next talent show at his middle school. He has recently joined the Special Olympics track and field team with his fellow classmates. He has also finally showed an interest in our family dog, with whom he engages daily—he even dabbles a little in training the dog with simple commands around our home. Puberty still evades us, but I know it's coming. I am terrified about what it will bring, but I am already mentally preparing myself for the storm and tapping into my resources.

If there is one piece of advice that I can pass on to you, it's to not lose yourself. Autism will consume you, and not always in a good way. It's all about finding balance and support in those tough early years, and remembering that if you don't take care of yourself, you will never be well enough to take care of your family. I know this for sure because I experienced it firsthand; my husband and I almost lost each other along the way. Take the time to connect with friends, and use your family or sitters to watch the kids as you go away for that long-overdue trip with your husband. Have a glass of wine now and again, and when it really gets tough, just breathe. This too shall pass, and brighter days are to come. This I can promise you.

Most importantly, when your journey is over and you have accomplished the unthinkable, pay it forward. Your journey is not only about paving the way for your child, but also about paving the way for the other families that follow you. It's your duty to help those families avoid struggles like yours and to not waste endless hours online searching for the right protocol, or doctor, or therapy that will help further along their child. It is in that moment that you pass the torch and inspire the warrior mom within all of us to move forward, to press on, to fight until you win, and most of all to spread hope. A hope that only you can offer because you have lived it, believed in it, and can now see it and hold it in your arms as it smiles back at you. So eat, pray, and sleep hope, my friends, and one day you and I will cross that finish line.

28

Guru Girl
Answers Are Out There!

As I sit on the bleachers next to the BMX track, I watch my son ride his bike and see him listening to his coach. I am in awe. He's only six years old.

I sit and reflect on the past six years of his life, and it all feels like a much longer period of time. How did my son, who was born premature at twenty-six weeks and diagnosed with autism spectrum disorder at the age of three, become this strong, determined, six-year-old boy I see before my very eyes? My answer? Biomedical intervention healed him!

Anthony's birth was not what you would call a glorious affair. During my pregnancy, at twenty weeks, Anthony's twin sister, Hailey, passed away. My OB/GYN and other medical staff tried to keep me from going into preterm labor. But at twenty-six weeks, my daughter was stillborn. Anthony, however, decided to do things his own way (as he does to this day) and stayed inside me for four additional days. Yes, my twins have different birthdays. Anthony was born via emergency C-section, weighing 2 pounds 3 ounces, 14 inches long.

His NICU experience lasted for ninety-one days. He had a grade 1 brain bleed, PDA ligation surgery at one month old (surgery by your heart), and seizures; his heart stopped beating a few times as well. He ended up coming home on oxygen and had an apnea monitor for his first eight months of life because 80 percent of his lungs were scarred. Despite all these complications, we were forever hopeful about the future Anthony would have.

The first year of Anthony's life was consumed with doctor's appointments and therapy sessions. Because he was born three months early, he was already considered a high risk for developmental delays and long-term health problems. The first week he was home with us, we started physical and occupational therapy. It was at that point that I figured out that I was not only going to be my son's mother, but his medical advocate/in-home nurse as well. I learned how to change out an oxygen cannula and apnea bands, how to feed a child who has a very poor suck/swallow reflex, and how to do physical therapy exercises with a child who is incredibly floppy because of low muscle tone. But even with the extra stress, I always looked into my son's eyes and thought, "You are my hero! You are strong, determined, and amazing! I know there is nothing out there that you won't overcome."

When Anthony was two, I became concerned about autism. He had caught up with all of his physical milestones at the time, but he was very behind in speech. At fifteen months old, Anthony had started to babble and had a few words. But as time went on, his words disappeared, and his babble turned to humming and grunting noises. He sounded as though he had duct tape over his mouth and was trying to speak through it.

Anthony began speech therapy, along with occupational therapy to help his fine and gross motor skills. He was diagnosed with speech apraxia and sensory processing disorder. Along with not being able to speak, Anthony also started drooling. Whenever he got excited, overstimulated, or touched a texture that was new to him, the drool would start flowing. He started rubbing his head on the carpet and pushing his body into people. He also started hoarding food in his mouth, and, while eating a meal, he packed his mouth full of food until he looked like a chipmunk.

As months went on, the issues started stacking up. There was talk of ADHD, OCD, and, of course, the conditions he was already labeled with—apraxia and sensory processing disorder. Each evaluation Anthony had was worse than the one before. No progress was made.

On Anthony's exit evaluation from the Regional Center, he was a year behind in speech as well as gross and fine motor skills. I vividly remember sitting in my car reading his evaluation report, with tears flowing down my cheeks. The therapy that all the doctors had pushed for was not helping Anthony. Not one bit. Something had to change! Therapy was not enough! There had to be something else going on inside my little boy. Something his current doctors were missing.

Soon after this, I spoke with an online friend I had met through YouTube. Her son was a surviving twin and had been born premature, like Anthony. She told me about biomedical intervention, DAN! doctors, and probiotics. She told me how DAN! doctors were treating the underlying medical reasons for autism spectrum disorder. The more she spoke, the more this sounded like what Anthony was dealing with. The very next morning, I found a DAN! doctor and made an appointment.

While we were waiting for Anthony's appointment date, I started him on probiotics. The first week he was on them, he spoke ten words! And for the first time in his life, he was able to repeat these words over and over! As the weeks went by, my formerly nonverbal son gained new words every day. He was able to say "outside," "car seat," and "sissy," and his list of words kept growing every day! I was shocked and in disbelief! Why? Because after two years of intensive speech therapy, my son had not gained one word. But after a week on a simple probiotic, he gained ten words! I felt hope and began thinking that biomedical intervention was exactly the treatment that would heal Anthony.

That first year of biomedical intervention was intense. I could never downplay that. Anthony was diagnosed with autism spectrum disorder, many food allergies, high yeast levels, mitochondrial dysfunction, methylation issues, oxidative stress . . . the list just went on and on. While I was overwhelmed with the news, I had hope, because we could fix these issues.

Life changed for my whole family that first year. We had to adapt to Anthony's new dietary needs. Not only did we have to go gluten- and casein-free with him, but we also had to avoid thirty other food ingredients, based on his Alletess IgG and IgE food allergy test results. After we received Anthony's Genova Diagnostic NutrEval Organic Acids Test results, which showed he had many vitamin deficiencies, high yeast levels, and inflammation, we started Anthony on many supplements, including a stronger probiotic with S. Boulardii (a good bacterium that kills yeast), omegas that would help with inflammation, Vitamin D, methyl B12 injections, and TMG to help him with his speech.

Anthony's recovery started right away. It was obvious that biomedical intervention was helping. His speech was growing by leaps and bounds. Even his speech therapist was amazed. She mentioned that whatever we were doing, we should keep doing it! After a few months of biomedical intervention, Anthony's sensory issues improved as well. He stopped drooling. He stopped rubbing his head on the carpet and pushing into objects. He even started feeling differences in temperature for the first time in his life. I remember him running to the refrigerator and saying, "It's cold, Mommy!"

Anthony's gross motor skills improved, too. At three and a half years old, he jumped for the first time. He learned how to do somersaults, kick a ball, and ride a balance bike. His fine motor skills improved so much that a month into biomedical intervention, he no longer qualified for occupational therapy.

His speech therapist advised putting Anthony into a typical developmental preschool to see how he would do. So at the age of four, he was enrolled in school. I was nervous, but I found a preschool that had warm and loving teachers. The students were very friendly to Anthony.

As his speech continued to improve with the help of TMG supplements, his confidence soared. For the first time in his life, he knew that people (besides his mom and dad) understood what he had to say. He made his first real friend and had his first real play date that year.

At four and a half, Anthony no longer qualified for speech therapy. I vividly remember that IEP (Individualized Educational Plan) meeting. I remember walking out with no written recommendations or goals. I remember crying happy tears as I walked to the car. It was a little over a year since we had started biomedical intervention, and I knew that's what we had to thank for this moment—the moment that my son became therapy free!

The past two years have all been about maintenance and refining Anthony's biomedical plan. As his body has healed, we have changed supplements. We have retested allergies and seen them vastly improve. He now only has one true allergy, which is gluten, and just a few food sensitivities. He used to have thirty.

We have fine-tuned Anthony's methylation protocol by running the genetic test called 23andMe. We found out that Anthony had two BHMT homozygous gene mutations and one heterozygous. This is the reason TMG helped him so much. We also found out that Anthony is heterozygous for the ACAT gene mutation, which is the reason for his mitochondrial dysfunction. We treat this with Cytotine and CoQH. And thanks to that, for the first time in his life, he is able to put some fat and muscle on his body and have more stamina.

Anthony is now six years old and in first grade. He is in a typical, mainstream classroom with no aide. He is age appropriate. He is reading, loving math, spelling words (even though he says it's not his favorite), and playing with kids at recess. He likes to swing on the monkey bars and go high on the swing set.

Anthony likes to play video games on his Wii U. He likes playing with Hot Wheels cars and Thomas the Tank Engine sets. He likes cooking and eating all types of food, especially Mexican food. He likes to visit his dad at work and "help out." He also likes to go to the mall. But Anthony's favorite thing in the world is to ride his bike.

So that's where I am today. Sitting next to the BMX track, watching my recovered son ride his bike, listening to him talk to his coach, watching him speed around that track just like his peers. We still are not quite a "typical" family. The four of us avoid gluten like the plague. I carry enzymes in my purse. I can talk for hours to a complete stranger about organic foods, GMOs, supplements, vaccines, DAN! doctors, and methylation issues. And if we go to a birthday party, I'm bringing my own homemade gluten-free cake; and no, my kids won't be drinking Coke.

Being recovered and on a maintenance protocol doesn't mean there are no little blips or setbacks. They happen, usually due to illness or diet infringements done by a third party. But the biomedical intervention has also taught me how to handle it all. It has taught me not to fear the "blips." I know that Anthony will never go back where we started out before biomedical intervention. Having that knowledge and the tools in your belt gives you comfort, confidence, and most importantly . . . *hope!* Hope that life will only continue to get easier and better for your child. Healing your child does not happen in a day, a week, or even a month. Biomed is a marathon! But is it worth it? With a lump in my throat and tears welled up in my eyes, I say, "Yes . . . my son is worth it!"

Update

Two years have passed since I wrote my original entry, and a lot has changed. Anthony is now nine years old and in the fourth grade. He loves playing basketball, reading, playing PlayStation games, doing math, and playing with his Nerf guns. He is still therapy free, no longer requires an IEP, and is still in a typical classroom setting with no aide. Recovered from autism? We can still say, "Yes."

I wanted to share with you all something that we discovered within the past year. Something that changed Anthony's treatment plan and ended up being a huge game changer in the process. This new information ended up taking the weight of the world off my shoulders for the first time in nine years.

So let's go back a bit . . .

When Anthony was six years old, he became very ill. After an emergency visit to the ER, he was diagnosed with lower lobe pneumonia. I had him out of school for two weeks, and, honestly, I had never seen him so sick from an illness. The doctors had him on antibiotics and Xopenex, but he still wasn't getting any better. After multiple visits to the pediatrician, she believed it wasn't so much Anthony's airways spasming; instead, it was most likely inflammation that was keeping his blood oxygen levels so low. She prescribed him the steroid medication Flovent. Due to his underdeveloped lungs, Anthony had been on this inhaler the first three years of his life, so I felt he would respond well to it. While his pneumonia seemed to vastly improve once we started the Flovent inhaler, a scary side effect occurred after three days of using it.

Anthony came to me one night and told me he was having a very difficult time speaking. He felt like his mouth wasn't able to say the words that were in his head. This really frightened me. I thought back to how Anthony had severe speech apraxia at a young age. I started to question if it was the Flovent inhaler he was on daily for three years. Perhaps this medication created the speech apraxia in the first place? Well, I wasn't going to take any chances. He only had a couple days left to be on the inhaler anyway, and Anthony was feeling so much better. I called his doctor and she said I could stop giving him the inhaler. His speech went back to normal within a few days. But after that bout of pneumonia, things just were not the same.

We started to see a different side of Anthony. He had severe mood swings daily—mood swings based on literally nothing. You could ask him a simple question like, "What would you like to eat for breakfast?" and his mood would swiftly turn from sweet and kind to a full-on rage. He said awful things. He talked about wanting to hurt himself, wanting to hurt others, wanting to destroy things. These rages would sometimes last for an hour or two.

There was no calming him or finding out what upset him, because like I mentioned, these mood swings were based on nothing to begin with. You could try calming him down, reasoning with him, punishing him, rewarding him for good behavior. But none of these methods worked. I felt like I was living with Dr. Jekyll and Mr. Hyde.

I contacted our DAN! doctor, whom we had worked with for years, and who had helped us recover Anthony in the past. But circumstances had changed. Our doctor's practice was now open only one day a week. My family had also moved, and we were now hours away from his office. Working together was difficult because of these circumstances. However, we tried to get around this by doing phone appointments. Anthony's DAN! doctor ordered some tests. We tested for strep, we tested allergies, we tested vitamin levels. Everything came back normal or unchanged. We tried changing dosages on supplements: increasing TMG, giving GABA, doing a yeast protocol. But nothing was helping. The only treatment that came close to helping with the mood swings and irritability was antibiotics. Yes, the dreaded antibiotics that destroy your gut.

When Anthony was on antibiotics, his behavior was better. His mood swings were not as intense, his irritability not as severe. But still they were present. Our pediatrician at the time recommended getting Anthony's adenoids removed. He thought perhaps the reason for his behavior was that he was having constant recurring sinus infections. His adenoids were enlarged and infected. This was confirmed by CAT scan and X-ray. And so with lots of hope, we had Anthony's adenoids removed. But as soon as he was off the antibiotics from surgery, his mood swings returned. I felt crushed and at a loss of what to do.

Neither our DAN! doctor nor our pediatrician wanted Anthony on antibiotics long term. I also knew antibiotics were never a solution, but emotionally I was at the point I could no longer cope. I was ready to lose it. I had panic attacks daily from the constant stress. We had been dealing with these mood swings for almost two years at this point, and I couldn't imagine living in this situation much longer. I felt like the rest of our family walked around on eggshells, trying to avoid Anthony's mood swings. Trying to avoid conversations. Trying to keep things "normal" for Anthony's younger sister, who was incredibly scared when her brother went into a full meltdown.

One night, around seven o'clock, Anthony went into a horrible rage. I can't remember what started it. I just remember him trying to hit me. He was saying awful things, scaring his little sister, who started crying. Anthony's dad stayed downstairs to console her. I got Anthony to his room and told him to calm down. He kept saying awful things, which was incredibly frustrating. I tried calming him down. I tried reasoning with him. I gave him punishments if he didn't stop this behavior. And again, nothing worked. You couldn't get through to him when he was in this state. After what felt like forever, I decided to leave the room, as he was screaming and kicking his door. At this point I would like to remind you this episode was all based on NOTHING! One second he was fine, and the next he was in an all-out rage.

I went into my pitch-black bedroom and flopped down on my bed. I stared up at the ceiling and just started crying. I couldn't do this anymore. I couldn't deal with this every day, sometimes multiple times a day. This wasn't exactly normal. There had to be a reason this was happening to him. This wasn't his normal personality. Yet, in the back of my mind, I knew it was something that had always been there. I had remembered similar behavior when he was little, after his naps. As I looked up at the ceiling I prayed to God to help me figure this out. To help me see what I wasn't seeing. Because after all, bio-medical intervention has taught me there is a reason for everything. But what was the reason for this?

I took Anthony in to his pediatrician and asked if he would run a complete autoimmune panel. There had to be something we were missing. He obliged and basically let me pick all the tests I wanted. I picked a ton of them! A few days (and $400) later, the results came back, and the only thing that was out of range was Anthony's TSH (thyroid stimulating hormone). It was elevated. I found this very interesting. Why? Because when Anthony was three years old, his TSH was elevated, too. I took him to a pediatric endocrinolo-gist back then. This "old school" doctor said that, while Anthony's number was elevated, I shouldn't worry. Yeah, well, I was worried *now*! Knowing this number was still elevated, I knew it wasn't just a coincidence. This number meant something. I knew it did. But even our pediatrician looked at it and said, "Don't worry. It's high, but not that high." I wasn't buying it this time. I was going to pursue this further.

The next day I knew what I needed to do. I needed to switch doctors. I needed to switch both our DAN! and our pediatrician. I had no problem leaving our current pediatrician. We had not been with him long. Luckily, I found an integrative pediatrician in our current city. She is supportive of all our work we have done biomedi-cally in the past. It is both a blessing and a huge relief to know that she is on our side.

However, it was an incredibly difficult decision to make about leaving our longtime DAN! doctor, who had been part of our family for four years. He was more than a doctor to me. He was a friend! He had been there at the time of Anthony's diagnosis. He gave Anthony his ability to speak. He helped us rid Anthony of all his sensory issues. He was the doctor that helped us get Anthony to a point where he was therapy-free. Going to another doctor almost felt like "cheating" on him. But I had to do it! I had to take that next step and go to the doctors that I knew would work together and help Anthony with his current issues.

So I messaged Dr. John Catanzaro via Facebook. Dr. Catanzaro is a naturopath with the company Health Coach 7. He is an author, speaker, educator, and leader in the genetic community. He has been using genetics in his naturopathic practice since 1996 with emphasis in immunogenetics. He is also incredibly knowledgeable when it comes to interpreting the 23andMe test.

Via Facebook, I gave Dr. Catanzaroa a brief summary of what had been going on with Anthony. Dr. Catanzaro said he would love to help, and that I should make an appointment with him. I booked the appointment online and sent Anthony's lab results, along with his RAW 23andMe data. A week later we had our first appointment, and it was life changing.

The initial consult with Dr. Catanzaro was everything I had hoped it would be. We went over Anthony's 23andMe results. We went over his labs from the past few years. At the end of the appointment, I had answers! The puzzle pieces were falling into place.

The first discovery was that Anthony's thyroid was in a downward spiral. His 23andMe test showed that, genetically, his thyroid was fragile to begin with. This information, along with his labs from when he was three years old and his recent thyroid labs, showed that he was experiencing hypothyroidism thyroiditis. We believe Anthony's thyroid was inflamed. The immune system created cytokines (cell signaling molecules that are triggered by an immune response.) Cytokines create inflammation and can suppress thyroid function. When Anthony was on antibiotics, the inflammation was reduced and thyroid function would improve. But the moment we stopped antibiotics, his genetically fragile thyroid would become inflamed again. Because of this new information, Dr. Catanzaro wanted to treat Anthony's thyroid with selenium and iodine. Before he started these supplements, we ran more blood work and discovered Anthony was low in both of these minerals. Selenium and iodine are both crucial to thyroid function.

What do I believe sent Anthony's genetically fragile thyroid over the edge? In my heart, I believe it was the Flovent inhaler that he was on daily for the first three years of life. This had a great impact on him and affected his speech. When Anthony was yet again prescribed Flovent for his case of pneumonia, it really sent him over the edge. Why? Because Flovent contains fluoride. Fluoride depletes iodine levels in the body. The thyroid needs iodine to function. When the thyroid is sluggish and not functioning well, you are dealing with hypothyroidism. What is one of the biggest symptoms of hypothyroidism? Moodiness, mood-swings, short-tempered behavior.

Another discovery made my jaw drop! But when I think about it, it makes complete sense. Anthony's 23andMe results and blood labs revealed an underlying metabolic issue regarding insulin and glucose production. Anthony's A1C results were only .3 points away from him being considered pre-diabetic! He was having a hard time with his blood sugar swinging from high to low (dysglycemia). Dr. Catanzaro believed that Anthony's mood swings and meltdowns were not only due to hypothyroidism, but also likely due to hypoglycemia—when your blood sugar becomes too low. This explained why most of his severe mood swings occurred first thing in the morning (before breakfast) and right after I picked him up from school, as he had not eaten in awhile.

I thought back to when Anthony was little and use to take daily naps. Anthony was an amazing napper and would usually sleep for three-hour-long stretches of time. However, when he woke up, he would go into a full-blown screaming tantrum. I always found these "tantrums" strange. He would wake up drenched in sweat. And while his eyes would be wide open, he acted as if he couldn't see you. He would scream and thrash his body all over the place. These episodes would go on for at least twenty minutes. Sometimes I would be able to get him to sip some juice, and this seemed to help. But other times, I could not calm him enough to drink. Eventually, he seemed to snap out of it and would have a snack. I used to joke that he was like me and just didn't wake up well from a nap. But now I know the real reason. After three or more hours without eating, his blood sugar was too low, and this sent his body into a rage and panic. All-over-body sweating can be a symptom of unstable glucose levels. Please, don't ignore it. I wish I had known better.

Dr. Catanzaro advised us to do the following in regards to this insulin/glucose issue:

1) Purchase a glucose meter, so I could monitor Anthony's glucose levels and figure out his trends.
2) Start Anthony on a high-protein diet and to make sure that with every meal and every snack, Anthony was getting protein. This would keep his blood sugar levels steadier.
3) Dr. Catanzaro's last recommendation was to have the Courtagen test run on Anthony, as he believed there was an underlying medical cause to this blood sugar issue.

What is the Courtagen test? It is a saliva-based DNA test that identifies conditions based on gene mutations (mitochondrial disease, seizures and epilepsy, and neurodevelopmental disorders). Dr. Catanzaro hoped we could find out exactly what was going on with Anthony's insulin/glucose production so that we could treat it. Because of the Courtagen Care Program, we received this incredibly expensive test for free. I recommend looking into it.

While we anxiously waited for the Courtagen test results, we began the new protocol Dr. Catanzaro had put into place for us. Anthony started his selenium and iodine. We started the high-protein diet (also known at the Mito Diet). And we started monitoring Anthony's glucose levels with a glucose monitor. The results were amazing!

Because of the selenium and iodine supplements, the puffiness under Anthony's eyes, which he had had most of his life, went away.

We had always thought his eyes were puffy due to allergies. However, they were actually puffy due to hypothyroidism. His hair also seemed to get softer, and his overall mood seemed to improve.

I started including protein with all of Anthony's meals and snacks. I increased the amount of food I sent to school with him and also informed his teacher about the situation. She was extremely empathetic, as she has type 1 diabetes. She understood how important it was for Anthony to eat often and lets Anthony eat in class if he's feeling "low." She also has mentioned how much happier Anthony seems in class.

If I see Anthony acting a bit irritable, and I know it has been a while since he has eaten, I will test his blood sugar and usually find that it is low. He eats a high-protein snack, and within fifteen minutes he is a happy camper. It is amazing how much a diet change can affect a child.

When Anthony's Courtagen results came in, I was very excited. It was one of those moments where you feel validated. I did have a right to be concerned! My gut instinct was correct, and there was something medically going on that could be fixed.

As I mentioned earlier, Courtagen is looking for conditions associated with genetic mutations. So when I saw that Anthony had a few "hits," and what they were associated with, I was amazed. I have listed the mutations below and what they affect:

SLC25A10: Inhibition of glucose-stimulated insulin secretion (GSIS) by 5 percent to 69 percent. Courtagen and Dr. Catanzaro have recommended magnesium citrate, as it helps bump up blood sugar to avoid hypoglycemic lows.

ACADS: Associated with fasting intolerance. With this mutation, Courtagen recommends eating often and also taking riboflavin (B2). We have since started Anthony on this.

And another interesting mutation that showed up:

LRRK2: Associated with OCD and anxiety. Anthony has experienced OCD since he was very little. And while he does not have life-altering compulsions, he does like to sort things when he is very stressed, usually only when something scary is going to occur, like having dental work done. But most days he is OCD free. Courtagen recommends antioxidant therapy for this mutation. We are using CoQH.

The new protocols we have done with Anthony based on his 23andMe, Courtagen, and lab results have been wonderful! Anthony has reacted extraordinarily well. I know this is the case because, genetically, his body is happy with everything we are doing. There have been no bad reactions and no detoxing symptoms.

After two years of hoping, praying, and pursuing answers, we have finally found them. When I recently spoke with both Dr. Catanzaro and Anthony's integrative pediatrician, I asked them if Anthony ever really had autism. They both strongly believe that Anthony's "autism" was really symptoms of multiple underlying medical issues. In this case, it was his thyroid and his metabolic disorder that impacts glucose/insulin, along with other genetic mutations.

We have to always remember that autism is strictly diagnosed based on witnessed behavior. But the big question is, what is the *cause* of that behavior? What is the medical reason behind its manifestation? Until you know what that answer is, never give up pursuing it!

If you would like to read more about our biomedical journey, Courtagen, and 23andMe, please visit my website www.biomedheals.com.

29

Oracle
Enlightened

O RACLE (NOUN): ANY PERSON OR THING SERVING AS AN AGENCY OF *divine communication.* An oracle is someone who foretells the future, someone who has a deeper insight on what's to come than most people do. Perfect! My friend TEX from the original Thinking Moms' Revolution chose my nickname, and it is totally me. While I am not a psychic or a medium myself (working on it), I do have vast knowledge of the subject and have used it to help my child with autism heal. My book, *The Other Side of Autism*, is a channeled book in which a medium and a spirit artist collaborated with me to help solve the autism puzzle.

Now, don't roll your eyes and think that I am some airy-fairy freak. I actually was forced down the spiritual path and into the realm of mediumship as a way of healing grief after the sudden loss of my first husband twenty years ago. After my first-born son Trevor was diagnosed with autism at age three, I learned a lot about healing him through this type of communication from my loved ones (and others) in spirit. In fact, I first learned that he was allergic to wheat during a session with a psychic medium. After the session, I had him tested, and the results showed that he was indeed allergic to wheat, among many other things.

But let us start from the beginning. Trevor was born in 1998, at the beginning of the "autism epidemic." Now, when I say "autism," I mean regressive autism. The "not born with it" variety. It drives me insane that people can't figure out that there are different forms of what they are calling autism. I'm talking about sick children, not neurodiverse people. These are distinct things, despite the identical label. This distinction needs to be made so that we can treat the sick children and love the rest.

My son was by natural childbirth born ten days late; he had a perfect 10 on his APGAR at birth, and we were overjoyed to have a healthy baby (or so we thought). He was a blond-haired, blue-eyed beauty who walked and talked at nine months and met all of his developmental milestones early. I did everything to keep him healthy and happy, including vaccinating him. My ex-husband's parents were Christian Scientists and did not vaccinate their three boys because of their religious beliefs. When the subject came up, I remember telling my ex-husband that I thought it was "child abuse" not to vaccinate your children. I carry the burden of that choice and feel like the Antichrist for my uneducated decision. The pressure, fear, and threats from the medical community won me over: "Your kids can't go to a public school if they don't have their shots." (I later learned that this was a lie.)

When Trevor was between ages one and two, something changed. He stopped looking at the camera while I videotaped him; we jokingly called it the "Elmo Trance." He started walking on his tiptoes and lining up his Matchbox cars into elaborate patterns, getting very upset if they didn't touch. The language he had been picking up suddenly stalled. He understood over twenty words at nine months and used the words "mama," "dada," "dog," "car," and "what's that?"

He had sixty words at a year old. He pointed, played peek-a-boo, and was very physically strong and agile, with great gross and fine motor skills. He fed himself with a fork at his first birthday party. A year later, I was feeding him his birthday cake, or he ate it with his hands. How do you lose the ability to hold utensils? He started pulling people to get what he wanted instead of talking. We had no clue what was happening.

He started limiting the foods he would eat to only wheat and dairy products. He was bottle fed (stupid me, again) and very colicky, so we had to switch formulas seven times in fifteen months. I now know why he couldn't tolerate them, but I'll get to that later. He started waking up a lot at night and wouldn't take a nap unless we drove him in the car. He was very sensitive to his environment, but so am I, so I didn't find that very concerning. He didn't like tags on his clothes (nor do I); he covered his ears when there were loud sounds (I sleep with a pillow over my head to block out sound); and he smelled things (I smell all food before I eat it). I also walked on my toes as a kid and nicknamed myself "Twinkletoes," so I could even reason that one away.

But then he began to show some really peculiar behaviors that I couldn't reason away: he wouldn't walk on grass with bare feet, he always had to carry toys or other objects in one or both hands, he looked at things really close to his eye, moving them back and forth, he made "hand puppets" with his fingers, often looking at them out of the corner of his eye, he would freak out for no apparent reason, he didn't seem to feel pain, and he started humming a lot. During a Mommy and Me gymnastics class, he seemed more defiant than the other kids—he did not look at or listen to the instructor and just wanted to do his own thing (run around and jump on the trampoline). I wanted him to be a gymnast, like me. It didn't take long to realize that it wasn't in the cards.

I was eight months pregnant with Trevor's younger brother, Damon, when Trevor went in for his three-year check-up. When his pediatrician saw that Trevor's Denver Prescreening Developmental score was worse than the previous visit, she became concerned. I'll never forget the moment I asked her what she thought was going on with my son. Before she could answer, the room seemed to change. I felt like I was alone in a tunnel, and I heard the word "autism" in my head before she said it herself. Then the room returned to normal. I chalked it up to some strange pregnancy thing at the time. She referred us for an evaluation with a developmental specialist. On the infamous September 11, 2001, we had the evaluation that led to my son's first official diagnosis of autism. My world imploded and crashed down around me. These were very dark days: postpartum depression, newly diagnosed child, PTSD from watching young widows grieve on TV (I was widowed young before marrying my kid's dad), new baby, no sleep.

More dark days were to come. Like in most autism families, there were money troubles and fights, therapies, depression, grief, listening to a screaming child for hours, stress, helplessness, blame, anger, and unhealthy coping strategies. Like many other autism families, my husband and I divorced. Then we remarried, and ultimately divorced again.

When my son was diagnosed, there was no Facebook, TACA (Talk About Curing Autism), Generation Rescue, or TMR. There was no autism roadmap, so I had to create one for my son the best way I knew. No one was really talking about diets, biomedical treatments, or any of the other things that are popular now in the autism community. Parents truly have the best chance for recovering their children when they start early. My son was five before I even started the diet with him. He was suffering and still getting vaccinated for two more years after his diagnosis until I started figuring things out.

Trevor was evaluated by the school district at age three and started in a developmental preschool program, which included any child that was "developmentally delayed" and qualified for services after their evaluation. They wouldn't even call his condition "autism" then; it was referred to as "developmental delay" until he was six.

I will never forget his first day of school. I had just given birth to my younger son and was emotionally and hormonally spent. The only people I ever trusted with Trevor until then were my mom and my ex-husband. So, here I was, leaving him with total strangers. He was crying, I was crying, and I was trying to convince myself that this was going to help him, when all I wanted to do was whisk him away and run far, far away. I finally was encouraged by the teacher that he was in good hands and left. I ran to my car and called my sister in hysterics. I felt like the worst parent on the planet. It turned out to be good in the long run, but it was very traumatic at the time. I'm sure many of you can relate.

Once he started school, he got sick all the time because his classmates went to school sick. Parents had to work and had no childcare, and the immune-compromised kids like my son picked up everything that crossed their path. I remember him having numerous ear infections and being on a number of different antibiotics. I still kick myself for this choice.

Meanwhile, during every free moment, I read everything I could find in print and on the Internet about autism. My two early favorite books were *Impossible Cure* by homeopath Amy Lansky and *Unraveling the Mystery of Autism and Pervasive Developmental Disorder* by Karyn Seroussi. They jumped off the shelf at the bookstore. Based on the latter book, I began dabbling in the gluten- and casein-free diet, but it seemed too hard—I had to make everything from scratch or order it online, because back then, there weren't the options you find today in the grocery store. On top of that, Trevor wouldn't eat anything I made. I had briefly given up, until I had that reading with the psychic medium I mentioned earlier, who in no uncertain terms told me that wheat was making him sick and I needed to strip it completely; Trevor would eventually get hungry and eat. And he did.

My son was five at this point. Around the time I decided to give the diet another whirl, a friend with a gluten allergy suggested that we start seeing her doctor, which we did. He was an Integrated Medicine Doctor, a former MD turned DO, who used homeopathy and herbal remedies. He used a noninvasive form of testing for food allergies, pathogens, and toxins called EAV, or Electro-Acupuncture According to Voll. It is a machine that reads your body for imbalances. The patient holds a metal rod in one hand, and the practitioner has a pointer that touches various acupuncture points on the hands that gives a reading on a computer screen and tells you what is going on in the body. It sounds like hocus-pocus, but at that point, I didn't trust the people who got us into this mess to get us out, so I had to try something else.

I ended up doing the allergy testing on myself, Damon, and my mom as well. We started using allergy desensitization drops to hopefully get rid of our allergies. We also discovered through the EAV that Trevor had high levels of mercury, yeast, parasites, and clostridia difficile (from all the antibiotics). I also did a urine Organic Acids Test on him, which confirmed many of these things (I was still unsure of the accuracy of the hocus-pocus back then, so I needed a lab test to confirm). We treated the metals, fungus, and pathogens with homeopathic detoxosodes (homeopathic detox). We also treated miasms (inherited conditions) and tried a constitutional homeopathic remedy. My son was getting better!

We eliminated all of the foods he was allergic to. When we took wheat out of his diet, it seemed like he could feel pain for the first time in his life; he actually cried when he fell down. He used to wipe out and not even flinch. He said "too hot" when he put his foot in the bathtub. Things were happening.

I recently dug up the list of allergens that my son had at age five (I learned of more later on). Among them were banana, beef, chocolate, corn, lettuce, milk, sugar cane, wheat, yeast, spelt, gluten, chlorine, red dye, yellow dye, formaldehyde, hydrocarbons, MSG, phenol, sodium nitrate, tobacco smoke, wood smoke, numerous molds and yeasts, cats, dogs, histamine, house dust mites, and numerous trees, grasses, and weeds. My poor baby! Allergies affect people in different ways, causing a variety of symptoms. They put stress on the body and prevent it from healing.

Being the impatient person I am, I did not want to wait twelve to eighteen months to desensitize these allergens with the drops. A friend had told me about our new doctor's old business partner, who did a quicker form of allergy elimination called NAET (Nambudripad's Allergy Elimination Technique). It involved muscle testing to find the allergens and acupuncture for adults (or acupressure for children) to instantly and permanently eliminate the allergies. Count me in! We went to the new doctor. This was a big treatment for my son. I still didn't feed him the problem foods even after the allergies were eliminated, but it gave me some peace of mind in case he accidentally got something at school. I knew the acupuncture worked for me. I was able to eat dairy again, never had to take allergy medicine again, and was able to be around a cat without having an asthma attack.

This was the start of my conversion to alternative medicine. After some real research and soul searching, I also stopped vaccinating both boys. My younger son, Damon, was vaccinated until he was fifteen months old, and then I put a stop to it. Around a year old, Damon became very constipated, and I found out through our new doctor that he was allergic to milk which caused the constipation, in addition to many other things. Like his older brother, he also had candida (both boys were born with thrush due to antibiotics I was given while pregnant), eczema, cradle cap (fungus), parasites, and mercury. We detoxed him as well with homeopathic detoxosodes.

His old pediatrician, whom I fired, tried to tell me that Damon had asthma and wanted to put him on steroids and a nebulizer. Damon wanted nothing to do with it, and he did not have asthma. He was sick with bronchitis two weeks before and again two weeks after a round of vaccines. I have no doubt that if I had continued to vaccinate Damon, I would have two "autistic" children. His brother saved him by teaching his mother what not to do anymore. Damon is an honor roll student and very talented and athletic.

As the next few years went by, I learned more and tried many different treatments and therapies for Trevor. He steadily regained skills every year, but he wasn't recovering as fast as I wanted him to. I kept searching and trying new things. I used homeopathy for all of our acute illnesses. If there was something I felt was over my head, our doctor's program could pinpoint what virus or bacteria it was and treat it with herbal and homeopathic remedies, not antibiotics, which do nothing for viruses anyway. The only time I would consider seeing a traditional Western medicine doctor is in an emergency, like a broken bone or car accident. They are good for that.

When I did the sessions with the mediums for my book, I learned a lot about what happened to my son leading up to his decline, and also about things that would help him get better. Without giving it all away, I'll mention some of the things that came up in the sessions as factors that affected my son's health: my taking prescribed antibiotics and a painkiller (which was later recalled) during pregnancy for a respiratory infection, early cord clamping (which depletes oxygen), the vaccines, of course, especially the MMR (the rubella component is made from aborted fetal tissue), GMO food, wheat, pathogens, and nuclear radiation. (The medium actually predicted Fukushima before it happened during our sessions!) It was made clear that there was brain damage caused by vaccines and other factors.

Some of the things that were brought through that would help my son included nutrition—especially eating non-GMO food, HBOT (hyperbaric oxygen therapy, huge for him), alkaline water (we have a Kangen water machine), and much more. After his first forty "dives" of HBOT in the hard chamber, he started waving to his friend at school and saying, "Hi, Austin." He also started buttoning his own shirts and putting on his own socks. Hello, small motor skills! He improved with everything I tried that was mentioned in the channeling sessions.

I believe that GMOs in our food supply are a very overlooked causative factor for autism. A lot of new information is coming out now proving the connection, including Stephanie Seneff's work. She is a senior MIT research scientist who says that the autism rate will be one in two by 2025 if things keep going the way they are; she argues that glyphosate (Roundup) and aluminum (in vaccines) are partly causing the spike. My son, born in 1998, was formula fed. The GMOs were added into milk first, starting in 1996. Then they made their way into corn, soy, cottonseed, sugar, and canola. What is in baby formula? Milk ingredients, corn syrup, and soy. Frankenformula. My son changed from formula to formula, tried soy and cow's milk, and was intolerant of all of them. It was the GMOs.

The built-in pesticides in GM corn are meant to rip open the stomachs of the insects that eat it. What do you think it is doing to a newborn with a compromised immune system? Leaky gut, anyone? Other GM crops are "Roundup Ready" and engineered to withstand the herbicide Roundup (glyphosate). Roundup has been linked to many health issues, including autism.

Children's first foods are full of GMOs and wheat (another poison).[1]

I also tried the most advanced form of biofeedback, called the Diacom, which is similar to EAV and Quantum Biofeedback (which we also tried). They all read the body energetically for frequencies that match diseases, pathogens, and toxins. The Diacom is a Russian technology that was developed for and used in the space program to diagnose and treat the astronauts. Only a few practitioners in the United States have it. Using headphones, the computerized program "scans" your body and compares the frequencies in your body with the frequencies of all pathogens, toxins, and diseases; it can even tell

---

[1] Jeffrey Smith, who directed *Genetic Roulette*, has a lot of information on the connection between GMOs and autism on his website, www.responsibletechnology.org.

you what organs are affected. It can also reverse the frequencies and treat the person, as well as make a water-based remedy with the correct frequencies in it. It has been very enlightening and validating, to say the least. Things that came up in the channeling sessions came up in the biofeedback sessions.

During one session, we found an intestinal infection, and the pathogens that came up were the specific parasite species we had been treating, along with *Borrelia burgdorferi*, the bacteria that causes Lyme disease (many children with an autism diagnosis have this), and Epstein-Barr virus. Trevor was treated with the frequencies and later that night, and for the next few days, he had a red rash on his hands and feet. It was a viral detox, brought on by the energetic frequencies. Homeopathy is also energy medicine. So are Reiki and Reconnective Healing, which I also learned to do for my son. We also use essential oils and flower essences. Yes, I'm the one that's "out there." Our kids are exquisitely sensitive, and I find that these things work for him. There is more than one way to skin a cat. Frequencies can heal.

I recently requested copies of my kids' medical records from all of their past doctors. I almost didn't want to look at them, especially Trevor's. Peeking into the past was a painful proposition. What stood out? Vaccinations every few months (thirty-four total), numerous antibiotics for ear and respiratory infections, including Cefaclor (in utero, in addition to Darvocet, the recalled painkiller), two rounds of Amoxicillin, two rounds of Zithromax, two rounds of Augmentin, and Cefzil. There were other medications, including Mylicon drops for gas, Nystatin antifungal for thrush, and later on Nystatin cream for a rash behind his knees. This was in the first three years of his life! I cried reading the doctors' notes.

At the same time, many of the doctors' comments were on how well Trevor was doing, how advanced he was, ahead of schedule . . . then it all went south. One startling thing I noticed in the records was that my younger son, who I thought didn't have an MMR vaccine, actually did, along with the DTaP the same day. I was mortified! Those were his last vaccines. He was very sick two weeks later, just before I left the practice and ultimately turned to alternative medicine. I also noticed two "Refusal to Vaccinate" documents that I had signed! I was wising up! Back in 2004. See, I am an Oracle . . .

So, where is my son today, you ask? Is he recovered? Has he reached the Holy Grail of autism? No, I cannot claim that. But he is the best he's ever been. He is in a private school without an aide. He is verbal, but limited. He can ask for what he wants to eat and do, but he won't ask me how my day was. He can read, write, do math, and type. We can take him anywhere now, and he loves going places. He is becoming more and more independent, trying to do everything himself. He is affectionate and tells me he loves me, which is music to my ears. His laugh and giggles light up the room, and everyone adores him.

He is still recovering. There is no time limit on that. People recover from debilitating injuries and illnesses all the time. A lot of damage has been done to these children at a critical time in their development—from things this planet has never seen before, I might add—and it's not always an easy fix. I will never give up helping him be the best version of himself and trying to get his body free of things that harm him.

What is the future that I see for our kids and for humanity at large? Even though it seems like an effort in futility right now to fight the powers that be, I do see a brighter future on the horizon. It will be the next generation—their generation, especially the siblings. My generation is mostly a lost cause, unless they are personally affected, a group that is growing exponentially. And pretty much forget my parents' generation, unless they are autism grandparents themselves.

Try to convince someone to stop eating food they have been eating their whole lives (that is now poison to which they are addicted). Gotta have that fast food, no time to cook. Try to tell someone completely indoctrinated into the medical mafia that there is another way to heal. They won't listen; doctors know best. You're a "quack" if you look into other methods of healing, which were actually around for thousands of years before this messed up system of medicine hijacked ancient healing modalities.

"Science" proves it, don't you know? Selective science maybe, paid-for science, tobacco science. There are studies that show what is happening to our kids, but when people don't have critical thinking skills anymore and won't even read the other side, it makes everything that much more difficult. It is going to get worse before it gets better. It may seem like the modern-day David vs. Goliath, and it truly is. But truth will prevail, it always does.

And people are waking up from their slumber; our kids are the catalyst to that. Because of our love for our children and having witnessed their regressions, we are tearing down the old, broken systems in medicine, government, food, and education. We are exposing the corruption, and they are scared. There is power in numbers, and ours are growing.

It is often hard to see the forest for the trees. It is easy to be angry and unable to see the big picture. In hindsight and through insight, I can see the good that has come out of what happened to my son. If he didn't have "autism," my family would still be eating and injecting poison, slowly doing who knows what to all of our bodies. We are literally human guinea pigs right now. Because of Trevor, we only eat organic, non-GMO, gluten-free food. Yes, it's challenging, but it's worth it. We would still be taking pharmaceutical medicine, which merely serves as a Band-Aid, and not getting to the root of illness. We have rediscovered ancient healing modalities. Everything that we put in or on our bodies and in our home has changed. We are all planting seeds in others and leading by example. Sharing our stories will prevent some of the lemmings from jumping off the cliff. Our children who were harmed are going to lead the charge, through us, to change the world for the better.

Update

A little update on what has transpired since I first wrote this two years ago. Trevor started having grand mal seizures at fifteen. He is now seventeen. I won't go into all the details, because I will tell the story in the TMR book on puberty, but essentially, he has had a grand mal seizure roughly every two months for the past two years, and it has been the scariest thing about the autism journey for me. The worst one was when he was in the HBOT chamber and I was outside and couldn't get to him. I thought I was having a heart attack.

We recently saw a board-certified chiropractic neurologist who did some bloodwork that showed that Trevor still has a leaky gut, even with his dietary restrictions. His body is having an autoimmune response to the tight junctions in his gut, which in turn causes an autoimmune attack on the myelin sheath in the brain. Leaky gut, leaky brain. The doctor also did a diagnostic visual test that could determine, based on how Trevor's eyes tracked and moved in response to certain stimuli, what parts of his brain are weak. How to fix it? Further dietary restrictions (basically Paleo—only meat, fruits, and vegetables, and no grains or nightshades), a few gut-healing supplements, and targeted brain exercises to strengthen the weak areas.

I learned that healing works in reverse as well. You don't have to start with the gut to heal the brain. You can heal the brain to heal the gut. We are just starting on the protocol, but I am very hopeful and feel that we are in good hands. The doctor feels that the seizures were caused by inflammation in the brain, and the new diet is anti-inflammatory. Diet is so crucial. Seven months seizure-free so far. A few times, he had two in one week. There is always more to learn, and I trust that the Universe will always bring us the right people with the right information to take Trevor where he needs to go next on his healing journey.

30

Karma
Leave No Stone Unturned

I AM CONSIDERED A "STAY-AT-HOME" MOM, WHICH IS IRONIC WHEN you consider the fact that I drive my four children, two twin boys and two girls with different needs, a minimum of sixty miles each day to two different schools, and that we spend upwards of three or four hours per day on the road.

In February, our drive changed after one semester of first grade, forty hours of Individualized Educational Plan meetings with our public school, and a few lawyers to haggle over the specifics of what is needed for two nonverbal children with severe autism to access an education. This started when the boys were three, and it took another five years to learn how little educational time one of the boys was receiving in the course of the day by the time first grade rolled around, which at this point was one hour out of a six-hour day.

During this year, the problematic behaviors that had been increasing for both boys since age three and the first year at public school had become a problem the teachers simply were not equipped to handle. I received reports of speech-generating devices being thrown and smashed, shoes tossed, and one boy would start crying and hitting himself in the head when his brother made any noise that irritated him. We had separated them this year, but even if they were in the gym or lunch room at the same time and he heard his brother whine or cry, he would have a meltdown. At home it was difficult to have one child that would throw himself down screaming if you tried to put him in the car to go to school, and who refused to wear a seat belt to the point where we applied for a grant for seat harnesses, which made him even more anxious, causing him to kick the windows of my car and try to escape. I had to repeatedly pull over to make sure he wouldn't hurt himself trying to get out of the straps.

Finally, my twin boys' names came up on what seemed to be the permanent waiting list for multiple services at our local autism center. We had already spent two years at this location in feeding therapy, parent training for feeding and behavioral strategies, and behavior intervention training for me and all four kids as a group. Now we're going back for intensive ABA (applied behavior analysis) therapy five days per week, as the boys have continued to struggle at school and at home. I had to withdraw them from school after working so hard to determine the cause of their lack of progress.

I have been the parent member of IEP teams for four children since 2009, when the twins entered the public school system in a self-contained classroom, which is the opposite of an inclusion setting with typical peers. The typical class size was about six kids with behaviors and needs of varying severity. Students had opportunities for exposure to regular classroom children at the school library, art activities, and in the lunch room. For me, being the parent member of the IEP team meant hours of preparation, pouring over each year's goals and data to see if progress had been made. This is just the tip of the iceberg of all that being a member of the team entails: weeding through reports, data, and evaluations, all while integrating a speech-generating device to facilitate development of their communication skills.

Our meetings were a stressful gathering of sometimes more than ten people sitting opposite our lawyer and me; meetings sometimes lasted six hours. I had to have a separate meeting for each child or I would get so overwhelmed I would miss details and mistakes would be made in the IEP, which is a legal document that needs to be accurate. I find it hard to express the extreme amount of stress and anxiety I felt when I had to approach a room full of people and repeatedly ask for increases in speech therapy for a child who lost the only ten spoken words he had, or for more occupational therapy for eight-year-olds who could barely write more than their names, and for ABA—known to be an effective method of teaching children with autism one on one—that the school district refused to provide.

The boys, soon after their autism diagnosis at age two, started a program and research project at our state university. It trained parents to teach their toddlers to use a speech-generating device. This can be an app on the iPad, such as Proloquo2Go, which uses symbols paired with words that, when touched by the child, generate a voice that speaks the word. The child can be taught to use it to request items and eventually build more complicated sentences. We started on a simple eight-panel device with large pictures with words, teaching the boys to request food. By the time we finished, they graduated to a GoTalk 20+, a green plastic device where I recorded my own voice. It has twenty words to choose from and now also exists as an app on the iPad.

The fact that they were able to not only learn how to communicate but progressed with each new device was a turning point for me. I had been told they had such low IQ scores that I wasn't sure that they could ever learn anything. By first grade, they had an expensive touchscreen computer device that they were supposed to have with them at all times. All people in their environment were supposed to use it to model communication skills, but this was a complicated process made difficult because staff needed more support in learning how to use it themselves. Imagine how difficult it must be to not only have limited verbal communication, but also have to learn the equivalent of another language, navigating through multiple screens to be able to ask for something that the average person just has to open their mouth to do; many people do not truly know how to engage. It is isolating and difficult.

Our commute begins at 7:00 a.m.; stop number one is Hazel's school. Our middle child—a four-pound preemie born at thirty-two weeks—she miraculously only stayed in the hospital for a week under the bili lights for jaundice. She was a tiny red doll, but she needed little medical intervention, which was a relief.

Before Hazel's second birthday, she was evaluated for speech delays by the state Early Intervention program therapists because she had only a few words by then, but they declared her "within normal limits" and denied services. I dismissed her sensory-seeking tactile issues, such as constantly needing to touch furry and squishy items, and her odd walking as imitation of her younger brothers, who displayed many behaviors associated with autism, such as toe walking. Hazel was kept on the vaccination schedule, as she was about to enter a preschool program that required them. Red flags continued as she entered kindergarten. She was sent to the principal's office the first month of school, because her teacher thought Hazel's refusal to join the group in circle time or leave the sandbox full of sensory input were defiant behaviors.

I was so wrapped up in IEP meetings for her siblings that I was completely caught off-guard when the school contacted me. They had the district autism specialist observe Hazel and her older sister Irene, who then identified them both as possibly having Asperger's syndrome, which had never occurred to me. Talk about being blindsided. Now in fourth grade, Hazel is struggling to find her place in the regular classroom. She loves cats, requires constant sensory input, and will only talk about her favorite online game to the point of driving her sister to shout "That's enough!!" at the top of her frustrated lungs. It gets very loud in our car, and between all the ruckus and the boys constantly unlatching their seat belts, it's a wonder we don't all have PTSD. On second thought, we probably do.

Our older daughter, Irene, is dropped off next at her charter school a few miles away. A fifth-grader full of humor and artistic talent, she has struggled the most as the oldest sibling of two younger brothers and a sister on the spectrum. A few weeks after being discharged from the hospital for E. coli poisoning in 2007, she started a pre-K inclusion program at a local university autism center, where college students are trained to work with ASD kids in the classroom. Her brothers were diagnosed a few months later; somehow it must have been on my radar subconsciously that we would need their help. We kept her on the recommended vaccine schedule in order to attend school, despite the fact that she spent a week in the hospital after birth with a severe case of jaundice. Looking back years later, I believe the jaundice was a reaction to the hepatitis B vaccine. As a full-term healthy baby, she was readmitted to the children's hospital PICU after her pediatrician proclaimed her "orange enough to be placed on top of the Christmas tree" with a dangerously high bilirubin level at three days old. No one connected it to the shot, and I had no idea.

At age five, not long after Irene's hospital stay, I noticed she was blinking excessively and making small jerking movements and vocalizations. I brought her to the pediatric ophthalmologist, thinking there was a problem with her eyesight. The doctor proclaimed her vision to be perfect, prescribed drops for allergies, and, when I asked about vision therapy, told me it was useless. The vocal and motor tics remained, and at age six she was diagnosed by her pediatrician with Tourette's syndrome and ADHD. Having already experienced ASD with her younger brothers, the minute I saw she was unable to complete worksheets and exhibited handwriting problems in kindergarten, I started the evaluation process with the school. After she was observed by the district autism specialist in first grade, I brought her and her sister to the center for evaluation. I had no idea it was possible to have two more children with autism. It was something I had never heard of.

We were still trying to wrap our heads around all of the medical issues with the twins, who were diagnosed with autism in 2008. How can you have four children with developmental problems? Isn't it rare? Both girls went to evaluations at the same place, same time in 2010, but Irene came out with a confirmed ADHD diagnosis; the therapist stated that she had characteristics of autism but was not on the spectrum. Her younger sister, Hazel, emerged with the Asperger's label. You would think that we would be used to it by then, but truthfully it is always a shock to hear those words. With girls, it is supposedly unusual to identify it at such a young age.

Pulling away from Irene's school, we head to our third stop, the autism center. The twenty-minute drive is bumper-to-bumper traffic of college students, hospital workers, and CDC employees. Driving past the CDC, a gleaming fortress of solitude, while taking my twin sons to the autism center for behavior therapy is an irony that is not lost on me. My heart aches as I wonder why it has come to this. I am grateful for the opportunity for our boys to finally get ABA, but why is this the only way? Our insurance doesn't cover the therapy, neither does Medicaid; the school does not provide it.

Last year I went to the state capital with another mom in the boys' classroom to get the state representatives to hear a bill called Ava's Law, which provides insurance coverage for autism services in the state of Georgia, with ABA being the most important. After years of languishing in committees, with politicians blocking it for fear of raising insurance premiums for constituents, this year the bill was finally being heard. As we were starting this new treatment program, Ava's Law finally made it through the state senate with a unanimous vote, but with an age cap of six and a behavior therapy coverage cap of $35,000. Ultimately it was not passed by the House due to the objections of a few lawmakers, one of whom has a major insurance company headquartered in his district and has vowed to never vote for it. Turns out, it would raise insurance rates an average of fifty cents per month.

Having back-to-back pregnancies, I was an overwhelmed mother of two toddlers when I became pregnant a third time. It was a high-risk situation that I was not ready for—what if it resulted in another premature birth? Only years after the fact did I learn how multiple medical interventions meant to save my newborns' lives could have contributed to their conditions.

In March 2006, my water broke on a Monday morning when I was twenty-five weeks pregnant with identical twin boys. I entered the hospital expecting to remain for a few months. Instead, they were delivered at twenty-six weeks via emergency C-section due to a prolapsed cord. Sometimes I reach in to a junk drawer and pull out a plastic sandwich bag containing a tiny diaper that fits in the palm of my hand, remembering the months we spent shuttling between hospitals, with their toddler sisters in tow, to visit our two-pound babies.

Before their birth, I was given antibiotics for strep, steroids to mature their lungs, and shots to stop premature labor. Examining my medical records years later, I found that a lung surfactant given at birth to prevent Respiratory Distress Syndrome has serious risks not revealed by the drug company, as addressed by the FDA in a warning letter to the manufacturer in 2011. It struck me that the drug trials on premature infants listed the many serious conditions associated with prematurity as side effects of the drug. Our sons, especially the most affected one, had almost every condition listed.

As I read this, I wondered how we could know if they were "born this way," or if all of the complications might have been caused by this drug. To stop premature labor, I was given shots of Terbutaline, which has since received a black box warning from the FDA advising against its use for prevention of preterm labor because it "may cause harm to the mother and/or the fetus." Terbutaline is also implicated in lawsuits that link it to the development of autism in twins. It crosses the blood–brain barrier in fetuses and can predispose them to developing autism; it can also increase vulnerability to environmental toxins. The more I read, the more studies I saw linking the drug's use to neuroinflammation, microglial activation, behavioral issues, and developmental delay.

There are many reports of antibiotics wiping out the good gut flora in newborns, especially those born via C-section, and I was on IV antibiotics for all three births, as well as lots of acetaminophen, which has also been implicated in autism and ADHD in recent studies.

Having twin micro-preemies in the NICU and going through all of the medical procedures and interventions brought new challenges to our family daily. Eventually, the boys were placed in separate hospitals several miles apart because one twin developed necrotizing enterocolitis requiring emergency surgery as he clung to life. Was the enterocolitis connected to the fact that he was tube fed milk-based formula as an underdeveloped newborn? The research I did afterward revealed evidence that premature infants are not able to process milk protein, which causes the intestinal tissue to die and rupture.

His brother got off lucky; he only had a chest tube and contracted a staph infection. I will never comprehend why our sick newborn, discharged from a four-month hospital stay after multiple surgeries and living on a diet of TPN and prescription hypoallergenic formula, was "caught up" on his immunizations before his release without our knowledge. Because we were unable to be in two places at once and also had no one to watch our toddler daughters, it was impossible to be at their bedsides for long. We did not know that things like multiple immunizations were going to happen because were not asked beforehand and were absent when they were administered.

Forty-eight hours after he came home, he was back in the emergency room, projectile vomiting and very jaundiced, something that was attributed to his medical and birth history. We weren't even told that we had to order special hypoallergenic formula from a pharmacy, so we'd mistakenly picked some up at the grocery store.

As a result, we find ourselves caring for our children in the aftermath of all of the chemicals, medications, vaccinations, genetically modified food, and environmental damage. I feel like I should have been wearing a hazmat suit instead of maternity jeans when I think of how my pre-pregnancy body was a toxic waste dump. I did not know a mouth full of twenty-year-old leaking amalgam fillings that needed to be removed could go bad and leak mercury into my body, exposing the babies to a toxic metal during each successive pregnancy. In the end, there are so many environmental factors, such as chemicals in our medicines, pesticides in food, and polluted air, that contributed to their fragile premature state, creating a perfect toxic storm that a two-pound baby could not withstand.

I believe that the damage done to our children in the form of autism and other childhood disorders is the result of decades of society and corporations not caring or not knowing about the effects their actions have on the environment and in turn on the people that come after them who reap the punishment for their carelessness.

Karma is the principle that what goes around comes around. The energy you put out into the Universe is returned to you. The concept of karma, in the most basic terms, is that every action has a result. One frequently hears "Karma is a bitch," meaning that all the wrong things people do will come back to get them in the end, a form of cosmic justice delivered by the hand of destiny. Karma has reared its ugly head and bitch-slapped us all as a planet. Only recently has a mainstream organization (the American Academy of Pediatrics) acknowledged that yes, there are environmental factors influencing autism, not just genetics. Unfortunately, most people don't realize that genes can be altered by their environment, including all the chemical insults that have become pervasive in everything that surrounds us. A saying that I heard at one of my fist autism conferences has always stuck with me: "Leave no stone unturned." I have held onto this over the years because I feel strongly that as a parent I have to research every avenue to make sure I am doing all I can for my children in order for them to thrive.

I keep putting out positive energy into the world that comes back to me in the form of hope. Hope should never be taken from anyone, yet it's taken away daily at the doctor's office, when they tell you there is nothing you can do for autism because, "We just don't know what causes it for sure." I call bullshit.

I think my biggest regret in life is that I have never had confidence. I relied on others to tell me what I should do because they were "experts" and I was "just a mom." While others were critical of Jenny McCarthy for going on *Oprah* and speaking about her son's autism, I watched intently. Then I dismissed her truth. Not because, as many people love to exclaim, "She's a Playboy bunny!" but because she was a mom like me, so what did she know?

I started looking at biomedical treatments a year after the boys' autism diagnosis in 2008. We were at the pediatrician's office for their three-year well check, and as I watched them screaming in their double stroller, the doctor told me to keep going to therapy and check back in with him in another six months, even though he never had anything new to tell me, nor did he offer any real help when he clearly saw my desperation. It was time to see what we could do, even when I knew we couldn't afford it, because it had to be better than doing nothing. Living on a single income with four small children, it was tough to make ends meet, let alone try interventions that were not covered by insurance and were also expensive and came with no guarantees. We had already filed for bankruptcy around the time of their first birthday due to financial struggles, the weak economy, and the copays for astronomical medical bills.

At night, I scoured the web for ways to fund treatments but came up short. I had visited the Generation Rescue site a few times and realized that Jenny, a fellow mom, had helped her son by doing the very things I was doing—researching. And then I saw it—GR was accepting applications for the first round of their Rescue Family Grant program. *Holy shit!* There was no way we were not going to get in on that! I filled out all the paperwork and nervously waited for notifications. I will never forget the day I got that call. I started screaming out of sheer relief. *Finally* we were going to get to try biomed for real.

While we have tried many interventions and found that my children often were "non-responders," I have never regretted doing the gluten- and casein-free diet. I feel that while they are not recovered, they would not be doing as well as they are now if I had not stuck it out and kept trying until we found our current regimen with the help of our new supportive doctor.

In 2014, we are six years down the road of our journey. I have been inspired by many in the autism community along the way; this is what has kept me going. Talk About Curing Autism, Generation Rescue, and the Thinking Moms' Revolution have been my anchors while I leave no stone unturned in getting to the bottom of my children's challenges. Sometimes I feel like these stones line the riverbed of our existence as the steady current of stress, illness, and isolation often rush over me and threaten to pull me downstream.

The other truth about karma is this: it is not predestined. You have the power to alter your course and therefore influence the outcome. Nothing is written in stone. I strongly believe that, although my children's progress has been slow and the fight has been exhausting, things will continue to improve. The more that individuals believe they have the power to enact real change, the more likely it is that change will come. Doing the research on medical and therapeutic interventions and being an informed parent without letting others pressure you gives you some control over how the events in life unfold instead of surrendering to someone else to make these decisions. It is up to you to enlighten yourself with the knowledge and confidence that you will make a difference and act accordingly. Remember, what goes around comes around.

Update

Two years have passed since I wrote this chapter. I now drive over 100 miles per day, but the boys are in a wonderful ABA program where my children have made gains in nearly everything. I have felt a sense of relief not having to be in endless meetings, fighting for the services that they need. They now are receiving those services in a private setting. I heard one of my boys, who had lost the few words he had for over two years, speak his first spontaneous sentence at almost ten years old. I have met many wonderful parents in the "parent room," a lounge created by the therapy center founders, who are also parents of a child with autism. They started their dream facility when almost none existed. The passage of Ava's Law in 2015 made it possible for many more families to receive these important services with insurance coverage, although the demand is overwhelming and there are not enough places to offer these programs. We are truly fortunate to be able to access them.

In March 2016, a friend and I visited the State Capitol, this time in support of SB145. This bill was to add seven qualifying conditions, including autism, to be eligible for access to low-THC cannabis oil that improves the lives of many patients but does not provide a recreational "high." Many children with autism also have seizure disorders and mitochondrial disease, and cannabis oil has been shown to be helpful in cases where prescription medications fail or the side effects are too strong. I know that my family would benefit from being able to use this oil and find it frustrating that it is not available in our state. I continue to support this cause for all children that need this medicine desperately and believe that it is the future of autism treatment that needs more advocacy and understanding.

The girls are now almost finished with sixth (Hazel) and seventh grade (Irene). They attend a charter middle school that is now in its second year. It was started by autism families. Over the past two years, the boys' behaviors have greatly improved. I am no longer worried about going out in public and fearing a meltdown. The boys have improved communicating their needs and can comply with requests, which is a big deal. Hazel has had many challenges, some undoubtedly due to the changes that come with being a teenager. This past year she basically slept through school and refused to do any work, prompting the staff to throw their hands up and say they could not force her. We had behavior challenges that have been very hard on me and her siblings, and I worry for her future while continuing to advocate for her to get the help she needs. She has shown an interest in photography, which I hope she continues, as she is talented. Irene has developed into quite the artist in many mediums and shows a desire to become an illustrator. We are very proud of our children and continue to be hopeful for their future as well as for progress in treatments for autism.

31

Rogue Zebra
From Blind Sheep to Rogue Zebra

"ABSENCE OF EVIDENCE IS NOT EVIDENCE OF ABSENCE." WHEN seeing a zebra, you might wonder whether it is black with white stripes or white with black stripes. Similarly, I often wonder if we are a spectrum family with additional medical issues or a complex medical family with autism-like tendencies in the older child and concerns for his sibling. Our diagnostic expedition started with a stroke . . .

"Negotiator" (as we would later nickname our son) was a reality check into parenting. He had clear likes and dislikes—he liked being held, for instance, and slept better with a tighter swaddle. Dad became proficient, and Negotiator would sleep through the night. He disliked tummy time, rolling in one direction, right arm tucked.

His milestones after six months came on the late side of the "typical" range. At his nine-month well check, I mentioned Negotiator's one-sided tendencies—he had been dragging his right foot when he cruised furniture. Then there was his preference for using his left hand. The nurse practitioner's interest grew: "How often is the hand preference, 50 percent, 25 percent?"

My heart sank. Hesitantly, I said, "90 percent." I cleared my throat and continued: "Ninety percent of the time, when we hand him something, he initiates with left." I learned that hand preference emerges between ages of two and four years; if it appears earlier, it should be investigated through Early Intervention and medically. The clues were so clear and obvious now that we were looking at the whole picture.

The neurologist met with us as a family, discussed paternal family history of "southpaws," did reflex examination, and ordered an MRI. In retracing the events and reviewing pictures, I have come to believe Negotiator's stroke happened between seven and nine months, six to twelve weeks from previous vaccinations. Negotiator was sedated, and a head MRI was done at eleven months. The diagnosis was suspected periventricular leukomalacia (PVL or ventricle stroke) or delayed myelination in left parietal lobe; eventually the whole thing was dismissed as "too vague, we won't ever know what happened." The doctor ended this appointment with phrases like "one-time event," "you probably don't even need to tell extended family," and "he might walk with a slight limp." We trusted his words to be able to live without the fear of what's next, and we trusted ourselves, having done what was expected by listening to doctors before and after our son's birth.

Eighteen months later, "Crash" arrived. Crash was a sleepy, quiet-dispositioned babe with porcelain skin and a head full of dark hair. Crash achieved her milestones—she simply had a poor quality to her skills. She rolled in one direction, proficiently. She wobbled her petite head, yet hated being on her back. She earned her strong tummy-time core, sitting at six months. She babbled and smiled at the slightest prompt.

But her arms and hands couldn't hold a bottle until it was half empty. At five months, her legs couldn't hold her own body weight (when supported). Later, she would try and try to rock back and forth, like she was trying to pre-crawl or pull to a stand, only to get frustrated and cry for a toy. We had concerns and weren't going to miss the signs again. Our pediatrician acknowledged our concerns and ordered an MRI of her head—the results were normal.

Crash started physical therapy at seven months for a "short episode of care, three to six months." Her core was strong, but her arms and legs were unsteady. Based on our observations and the PT's concerns, our pediatrician ordered an MRI of her lumbar spine; the results were normal. She continued PT for another six-month episode of care. Now eleven months old, Crash could pull up, her right foot planted, knee bent, and leg pushing up, while other leg tried to sneak in support; the time elapsed from the first pull up to standing for a few seconds on both feet was seven minutes. We continued PT for another three months. Crash was then discharged from PT, stepping independently for short distances at sixteen months old. Crash did not have a brain injury or lower spine injury to explain her hypotonia and gross motor delays.

Around two and a half years old, Negotiator began screaming for sixty to ninety minutes after being laid to sleep. He'd be alert, but not awake and responsive. The neurologist said it was night terrors. And we listened, again trusting his judgment. After eighteen months (and a broken collarbone from falling out of bed), we got a second opinion, and this doctor agreed with the previous diagnosis. When the screaming started occurring at nap time as well, our pediatrician said to get a third opinion at an internationally renowned clinic.

They did a full week of testing that produced few answers but did confirm seizures, so the doctors prescribed a medication. The medication helped his seizures and nighttime wakings, but oppositional argumentative behaviors and emotional tantrums increased tenfold. Six months after the first visit, I figured life could not get worse than where we were: stroke, seizures, ADHD, speech delays, and a four-year-old's tantrums of epic potential . . . and Crash with her own developing issues. We already had full-time sensory processing, behavioral, and rehab therapies, plus home routines that included improving specific fine motor or gross motor skills. These were not helping anymore. Autism—or whatever label the latest psychologist decided on to fit their agenda—was winning.

I had my own sensory processing meltdown, deciding Negotiator and Crash were going gluten-free for six months. Cold turkey. Crash didn't eat much table food, still preferring scheduled predigested formula in a bottle, at two years old. It was the only nutrition she didn't vomit daily. Suspect food went into the freezer or pantry. Milk and cheese were *the* favorite of Negotiator, however. We cut off casein two months into the GF trial. The peak of withdrawals occurred at the holidays that year. Life went from crazy days to living in each chaotic moment, focused on the unknown recovery possibility. Six months of a gluten- and casein-free diet gave us enough evidence of improvement to continue. He had no seizures in six months—he was still on meds, but there were no breakthrough seizures. There were also improved emotions, more communication, and more engaged activities out of his comfort zone.

We planned a trial of adding gluten again for one week, without telling the therapists (so that we could get an objective evaluation of any changes). It only took three days for the hand-flapping stims and behavior extremes to return; his OT asked what we had changed. Future diet challenges over the years reintroduced his complex partial seizures and emotional extremes.

Our initial success with GFCF led to additional biomed protocols with guidance from warrior moms who blazed the trail. Learning the signs of candida, then treating with olive leaf extract and probiotics. Food journals. Poop journals. Tracking activity and behaviors. Checking developmental progress on AAP and CDC charts. Learning lifestyle tweaks for phenols, oxalates, and other micronutrient food groups I'd never considered the existence of before 2005. Eliminating phthalates, chemicals, and cross-reactive foods. We were solving problems one or two at a time with lasting results.

Negotiator was stimming less, working for behavior rewards more. Crash stopped vomiting, finally. We turned that corner in 2009 and had no major changes to baseline for three years when the kids' issues began to shift back toward more medical symptoms (increased fatigue, dehydration episodes). Skills plateaued for both, but they were thriving and excelling in a virtual school setting, where we could work at their pace without distractions, illnesses, or bullies.

In 2011, Negotiator started a compounded mitochondrial cocktail, a combination of vitamins and minerals specific to a child's individual needs; Crash didn't tolerate her custom supplement cocktail. In 2012, we survived flu season needing only IV fluid support, without long-term hospitalization or regression of skills. Puberty also hit both kids, despite the three-year difference in age. In 2013, new symptoms continued to appear—central apnea requiring BiPAP (Bilevel Positive Airway Pressure) nightly and weaker respiratory muscles requiring HFCWO (a high frequency chest wall oscillator) added to the daily nebulizer protocol we had already implemented. Fatigue continued to progress; currently both use powered wheelchairs for community distances. They are facing more medical treatments than any child should bear, but they have far fewer than other Mighty Mito Fighters routinely have in their daily life.

In those same eight years, we have seen dozens of medical specialists, locally and across the country. Negotiator's stroke led to night terrors and seizures, after which his muscle weakness and fatigue would not improve. Crash was holding her own—a phrase I'd often use to describe her lack of progress. Their constellation of signs and symptoms—stroke, seizures, ADHD, hypermobility, muscle weakness, growth delays, sleeping ten to twelve hours, nutritional deficiency, Asperger's, verbal and oral apraxia, delays in gross/fine motor skills, receptive/expressive language delays, and social deficits—represents many possibilities, especially if the doctor excludes one or two symptoms.

Each new specialist added their perspective; some offered testing for a specific group of possibilities: Rett syndrome, congenital myasthenia gravis, spinal muscle atrophy, congenital myopathy, thyroid diseases, mitochondrial disease, fatty acid oxidation disorders, urea cycle disorders, osteogenesis imperfecta, Ehlers-Danlos, deconditioning (of muscles), and recently Charcot-Marie-Tooth disease. All of these lead back to clinical mitochondrial disease until another disease is proven.

Results would come back as abnormal but nondiagnostic (EEG, EMG, frozen muscle and skin biopsy, fresh muscle and skin biopsy, mtDNA and nDNA genome tests, MRI with MRS); sometimes there was a rare negative/normal (chromosome tests, complete metabolic panel, and other blood/urine lab tests). A buccal swab screening test came back confirming mito dysfunction at an over 90 percent deficiency: "Crash was significantly low, Negotiator was more extensively diminished." We have labs, physical history, and genetic findings to clinically support a probable mito diagnosis. Science is still unraveling DNA to make our diagnosis solid.

There is a Someecards meme that states, "A special needs Mom's research is better than FBI." That's me. I have no plans to be a doctor or other medical professional, but I do have a vested interest in my kids' health and wellness. Partly because of the early oversights and partly out of genuine curiosity, I still spend my late nights reading. I often read back through the extensive three-ring binders of clinical notes and ask questions or explore a new possibility. Maybe the doctors missed something—since food choices clearly improved outcome—maybe there's a new possibility, more ideas. I review clinical notes, looking for any new information about a mutation found six years ago—a lifetime in genetic research. I have found really awesome medical websites to help me fit our puzzle pieces together. I was gaining a greater understanding, that all of our kids' symptoms were metabolically driven. I narrowed my focus to metabolic processes (how protein, fats, and carbs are used, broken down, or stored) and mitochondrial disease (how food is converted to energy).

My knowledge—as well as our diagnostic expedition and non-pharma successes—set us up for suspicious doctors. You know the ones. They've had a one-hour lecture on mitochondria and genetics in four years of medical school. The proud, confident doctor who can see your red flags without gathering a ten-year history; who surely knows more from books or lectures that haven't been updated in the last five years; who observes the patient for clues, never talking to patient directly, and completely ignores parental insights. His/her perception is that parents are doing this "diet" because it's simply a trendy fad or easy and fun lifestyle. Heck, even the child's symptoms are seen as simply attention-seeking behavior.

Obviously, we would *choose* eight years of rehabilitation therapies, so our child could achieve age-level skills, only to lose those gains with the next viral illness. Clearly, we would *choose* special complex "diets" that exclude our children from family gatherings, school events, and virtually every major public facility. Who wouldn't? Please.

The reality is we make these choices and sacrifices so our children thrive and expect to do more despite what the poorly informed medical community has done to them. We didn't have children just to have them survive in mediocrity. Our children's bodies are failing them. We are competing in a race against time. They don't have the energy to live day to day like other kids, so how can they do more?

Mitochondrial dysfunction causes their behavioral, social, physical, and cognitive difficulties. We continue to need specialist support, so we chose a virtual mito doctor, who created a practice for mito patients with their needs in mind. She understands the travel limitations, the effort travel takes, and the expenses involved. She understands the frustration of waiting for science to catch up, the vagueness of labs, and the varied presentations within a family. She communicates that understanding. She validates our conclusion that the buccal swabs support our kids' symptoms and historically quirky labs. She is willing to support a probable mitochondrial disease, until there is a different diagnosis. She shows her support by listening and giving precise answers, even when she can't give a firm prognosis. She easily adapts her answers to your understanding—novice or late-night reader. She gives us peace of mind and confidence to continue this journey, guiding our direction while enabling us to *think* as parents, not solely medical advocates.

Unlike zebras, who are born with their stripes, Negotiator and Crash were not born with mitochondrial dysfunction, autism, or any inherited condition. Medical students are taught to diagnose by idiom, "When you hear hoof beats, think horses, not zebras." Same for non-thinkers. People see the white stripes, but not the black stripes or the skin underneath. People see the illusion of the able-bodied, healthy-looking kids. People miss the reality—kids fighting to live longer. Our expedition continues, seeking the distinction between the mimicry of the zebra's white stripes and the zebra's true black stripes. I am optimistic that their recovery will outlast my life-time. Negotiator and Crash will recognize the power in themselves to make choices and consider the consequences of those choices. Negotiator and Crash will think for themselves as children of the Thinking Moms' Revolution.

Epilogue

W HEN THE ORIGINAL MEMBERS OF THE THINKING MOMS'
Revolution wrote *Autism Beyond the Spectrum*, our goal was
to share our stories and inspire others to do the same, with the hope
of reaching every parent of a child with a developmental disability to
give them the message that they are not alone, and that there is hope
for their situation.

At the time, a not-for-profit organization to help families finan-
cially only was an idea, just as the book, now realized, had been an
idea the year prior. I am happy that Team TMR came to fruition and
that we can pay it forward in the form of granted funds for treatments for families that need help.

ShamROCK approached me about a year ago after reading
Autism Beyond the Spectrum with an idea that gave birth to *Evolution
of a Revolution*. She was inspired after reading our book and wrote
her own chapter. She added her chapter to the back of our book and
read it at her book club meeting. We blogged about it and encouraged others to do the same.

After the formation of Team TMR, we reached out to Thinkers
and asked them to donate their stories of recovery to a special text,
the proceeds from which would be used to fund our treatment grant
program. The response was overwhelming, and to keep the book
manageable, we had to take the request down after just one day.

That tells me our stories are a powerful tool to spread hope to other families who do not yet know that biomedical and alternative interventions can really work wonders on a child with autism. The recovery stories in this book happened. And recovery from autism continues to happen every single day.

I hope that you, our reader, will be inspired to write your own story. Share it with your family and friends, your book club, your bible study group, and your Bunco pals. Together we are changing course. Autism is not a jail sentence that ends in institutional living, as we are so often told by our neurologists. It is a toxicity problem that, once addressed, can reverse course. What are you waiting for? Get out there and change the world with us! To become involved with our mission, visit us at www.teamtmr.org.

Helen Conroy
Executive Director, Team TMR

Acknowledgments

W E, THE MEMBERS OF TEAM TMR WHO HAVE CONTRIBUTED to this book, would like to thank all of the thinking moms and dads that write blogs and web pages on social media sites, the brave doctors who have put their careers on the line for the sake of our children and their health, the politicians who are trying to change the ways of the government, the advocates who tirelessly work to pave the way for our children, and the educators, paraprofessionals, and therapists who took the time to care about and help our children.

There are certain organizations and individuals that have helped us on a profound level. They are Generation Rescue, TACA, Jenny McCarthy, Stan Kurtz, Autism Research Institute, David Kirby, AutismOne, Age of Autism, The Canary Party, Safeminds, Ginger Taylor, National Autism Association, Dr. Wakefield, Rob Schneider, and Aidan Quinn.

Whether we were introduced to the original members of TMR via their blog or their chapter in their book, we all agree we felt an immediate connection to one or many of them as we read their words, their stories, their inspirational messages. As we read the blog each day, we knew we were no longer alone on this journey to ultimate health for our children.

Through their written words, we were made to feel as though we were all connected, united on this journey of healing and hope. The TMR was and is a breath of fresh air in this community. We are so very proud, humbled, and grateful to work alongside these extreme warriors, and we are elated to be a part of Team TMR. Thank you to all of you for guiding us, for sharing your stories with us, and for taking us under your wings. Thank you for befriending us and showing us that hard work and determination can and will make a difference in our community.

About the Authors

Barracuda (Julie Clymer Pletner): I am a mom to an amazing nine-year-old girl who has taught me the true meaning of love through the journey of recovery, and a wife to a hands-on husband who shares my passion for recovering our daughter. I'm a family support coordinator at the Kennedy Donovan Center on Cape Cod, sharing information and resources with those in our community with intellectual disabilities. It is my dream job! There is nothing better than being able to pay it forward.

Beaker started her professional career in the lab as a bewildered chemist who often felt she was a round peg in a square hole. After her daughter's multitude of medical issues, she found out the exact reason she had that graduate chemistry degree and put it to good use as she set out to restore her child's health. Along the way she found her true calling: sharing her family's experience with other parents (especially mothers) and helping them improve the quality of life for their children by staying true to their guiding light . . . their God-given mother's instinct.

Bling (Heidi Scheer): I am a true girlie-girl who was raised in a house of boys. I am the mother of three incredible children and the wife of the most amazing man on Earth. My middle son is recovered from autism and is, by far, my family's greatest example of perseverance, courage, and faith. As they say, it takes a village . . . and I am here to join yours!

Chief (Jennifer Young): I am a Southern born-and-bred registered nurse and mom to Madison, who is recovered from autism. I have settled nicely into my crunchy-mom role after years of working to heal my daughter. If you need me, check the grocery store or my kitchen, where I whip up gourmet SCD cuisine. Just kidding, it's chicken and carrots.

Co-Pilot (Heather Jung): I'm a military spouse and mom to two beautiful children. My daughter, who's five years old, had autism and bowel disease. My two-year-old son is neurotypical. My husband is a pilot in the Air Force. He serves our country and I serve our family. Though he travels a lot, he is very involved in our daughter's recovery and we make all decisions together. As the military life goes, we find ourselves on the move a lot, and our lives can feel pretty hectic sometimes, but we always try to make time for the things we enjoy doing together as a family.

Cougar (Ginger Lee): I'm mom to four children: two boys and two girls, the oldest of whom is recovered from autism. A loyal friend, a loving mom and wife, and a lot of fun, I'm also fierce in my pursuit to right the injustice that's been done to a generation of our precious children. I will not stand idly by while our kids are being poisoned. This will end. I am the Revolution! You are the Revolution!

Creole Queen (Keisha Hertzock): *Rawr! I'm a tiger!* I'm a southern woman from Louisiana. God, family, good music, good food, big dreams, and red lipstick are everything to me. My six-year-old son has autism. My four-year-old son has autism and a digestive disorder. My two-year-old son is experiencing delays in his development.

Through it all, my faith remains strong. My six- and four-year-olds have made awesome progress and continue to shine, and my sleeves are rolled up as I'm working with my two-year-old. Prayer is my steering wheel! *Remain strong and keep hope!*

Crush (Shannon Strayhorn): I am a mom to two amazing little girls. Cali is my recovered eleven-year-old daughter who is going to change this world, and Melia is my eight-year-old daughter who is her sister's best friend and strongest advocate. In my home life, I am a silly, laid-back mom who has the good fortune of being married to my best friend. I celebrate life and love nothing more than family, laughter, and time at the beach. In my "autism" life, I am a feisty, sarcastic, common-sense thinker who is on a mission to *crush* the limitations placed on our children, *crush* the lies of these epidemics, and *crush* the people standing in the way of truth, hope, and healing.

Frankie (Andrea Frank Giboney): I'm mom to three amazing children who, along with my husband, are my heart and soul. At the age of three, my son was diagnosed with PDD-NOS, and we were told his future would consist of group homes or state run facilities. With biomedical treatment (and a lot of sweat, tears, humor, and love) he is now recovered. I tossed the rose-colored glasses, rolled up my sleeves, and made his recovery my mission. I hope his story can inspire others to do the same.

Green Bean Girl (Meadow Davidson): I am a Midwestern mom trying to adapt once again to Southern living. My oldest son is eighteen and has been on the autism spectrum since age two. My sixteen-year-old was diagnosed with sensory processing disorder, anxiety, and Asperger's. I worked as a special education assistant, but decided to teach my boys at home this year and we are loving every minute of it! We have a beagle, Maddy, and two cats named Aqua and Patches.

Guardian (Sadie West): I am a wife and a mom to ten-year-old twin boys. I have lived in the suburbs of Chicago all my life. I am a developmental therapist and autism education advocate. My mission is to teach others about the strategies that work best in our educational settings so our kids can be successful learners. I love spending time with my family and friends and need more time to do it!

Guru Girl (Kim Ruckman): I am a SoCal mom to two wonderful kiddos and wife to a very sexy software engineer. I volunteer my time as a grant mentor to Generation Rescue's grant program, and I am also the creator of *Biomed Heals*, a website that chronicles my son's complete recovery from autism. I'm a problem solver at heart and will never back down if I think something can be fixed! For work, I am a Beachbody Coach. I love working out in the comfort of my own home and helping others do the same. Fitness is my zen and what keeps me sane—which works out great, considering that 90 percent of the clothes in my closet are active wear.

Hoppy: I am a mom of two handsome little boys who light up my life (almost) every day! Proud owners of a brewery and farm-to-table restaurant, our family believes that nature knows best when it comes to our bodies and our foods. I focus on having fun with my boys and my work, and everything else falls into place!

Juicy Fruit (Joy Whitcomb): I am the mom to a beautiful eleven-year-old boy who regressed into autism as a result of the influenza virus (not vaccines) at age three. We have spent the last eight years working to get him back, and he is doing amazing. I work in corporate America by day and fight as a Mother Warrior by night. We live in Colorado and have three poodles that are our de facto service dogs.

Karma is "just a mom" to four kids and spends way too much time navigating their dirty minivan through the urban sprawl that is metro Atlanta. She proudly supports Generation Rescue in the role of parent mentor for their Family Grant program. When asked, "How do you do it?" her answer is simple: coffee, Belgian ale, and an odd sense of humor.

Lioness: I am a forty-something mom to two girls: a nine-year-old with Down syndrome and autism and a fun-loving and spunky typical five-year-old. Before having children, I dabbled in bellydance, Native beadwork, and Tsalagi (Cherokee) language lessons. I even considered going back to school to become a zookeeper. After the autism diagnosis, I became a Lioness, protecting and providing every resource I could to ensure recovery for my daughter. I also spent a lot of time wanting to "attack" the predators of Big Ag, Pharma, and Government for damaging our kids. But this last year brought some physical and mental changes that brought me 'round to myself and a lot of introspection. I renewed my love of Jesus and am providing for my own wants and needs. As a result, my whole family has been slowly transforming for the better.

Lone Star (Michelle Taff Schneider): I'm a proud Texan and a mother of three. My middle child, now five years old, was diagnosed with autism at twenty-seven months, more than a year after her initial regression. I have no shame in admitting that her recovery, in one way or another, has consumed my life. I have discovered a level of strength and determination I never knew existed within me, and the challenges have taught me so many things about her as well. Through this journey, I've met so many committed parents who also believe that autism is preventable and treatable, and I've made it my personal mission to support families and educate as many people as I can about the facts. I'm a founding member of and communications director for Texans for Vaccine Choice, and I've also assisted with research for the recent documentary film *Vaxxed*.

Monarch (Jennifer Swanson Collins): I majored in philosophy in college and still believe in questioning and examining all issues, arguments, and dogma. At heart, I am a humanitarian, a little quirky, and a dreamer. I am soft spoken with a permanent smile, but I am a fighter, fearless when it comes to caring for and healing my children. I am the mother to a set of beautiful and sensitive twin boys diagnosed with autism. The twins have a toddler-age sister who demonstrates symptoms of toxic injuries. She has been treated with natural supplements and diet since birth and is showing incredible healing. I feel my true purpose in life is to unite with other Thinkers and spread the *truth* and a message of hope. I believe our children's stories have the power to change the world!

Muscle Mama (Mary McKnight): I am a mother of two beautiful children, the oldest of whom is diagnosed with autism and hyperlexia. I love working out to stay focused and to never forget who I really am, and I love to educate people about autism and help families whenever I can. My favorite thing is hugs from my kids, because they are growing up so fast! My best trait is that I don't give up . . . *ever*. No matter how long it takes or how hard it gets, autism is going down, and I have the muscles to prove it.

Oracle (Laura Hirsch) has a B.A. in speech communications and is the author of three books. Her first book was an autobiography about her experience of being a young widow, which led to her investigation of mediumship as a therapeutic avenue for grief. She remarried and had two sons, the older of whom was diagnosed at age three with regressive autism. Her love and devotion to her son led her back to mediumship for answers from her loved ones in spirit and others on how to heal her son. She worked with a psychic medium and his wife, a spirit artist, and they extended an open invitation to the spirit world to help solve the autism puzzle. Her third book, *The Other Side of Autism: Famous Spirits Unveil Regressive Autism's Causes* *and Remedies*, is the culmination of their sessions. She is also a non-GMO advocate and is featured in the documentary *Genetic Roulette*. Her website is called *The Other Side of Autism*.

Phoenix (Lindsey Articolo): I was born again from the ashes of my life before autism. I am a mom to Ava, who is nine, and twins, Andrew and Ben, who are three. Andrew was diagnosed with ASD at twenty-one months. The best part of this journey has been learning to enjoy it. At the same time, it is hard for me to pretend much else matters besides our kids, who are so much like canaries in a coal mine.

Queen B (Christina Johnson): I am a tried-and-true Midwestern girl and a mother of three beautiful and precocious children, who are my everything. My ten-year-old daughter is diagnosed with autism, but we now also know about her many underlying issues that make up that diagnosis. I am constantly researching to find the best interventions and figure out a way to afford them all. Our daughter didn't make significant progress until she was seven years old, so I know there is always hope! I try to make it all work while juggling a full-time job and being a mommy and a wife. I have an amazing husband who supports my obsessive search for answers and an amazing support group of close friends (my Warrior Mom Tribe) who are there for me no matter what. Oh, and I like my occasional cocktail and ice-cold beer to take the edge off once in a while, too.

Rainmaker (Tyler Dahm) lives in Colorado and owns Pathways Integrative Wellness Center, where families living with autism and other chronic health conditions can go for treatment. Tyler is a Holistic Health Practitioner specializing in autism, cannabis counseling, genetic counseling, virology, and detoxification. She educates physicians all over the world on effective ways to treat autism. Tyler also presents at conferences nationwide and is known internationally as a detoxification expert. She has turned her story of loss into one of hope by working with Team TMR and the Stephen Dahm Autism Treatment Grant to offer help and resources to autism families all over the country at no cost.

Rebel (Mary Pulles Cavanaugh) is a mom of three girls. She became an avid researcher in 2008 by necessity when she began the autism journey that led her to awareness of the sick-care system that is so prevalent today. What keeps her focused is the knowledge that we are fearfully and wonderfully made. She is most proud of her upcoming book, *The Book On Greatness: How To Keep Shining Your Light*. Rebel looks forward to a future with natural healers of the mind and body, and many future travels discovering new places with her husband of twenty-nine years. Her current focus is on staying uncomfortable and manifesting change. Her website can be found at marypullescavanaugh.com. You can also find her on Twitter @max4metals.

Rocky (Nicki Di Bari Roxby) grew up in large Italian family and still enjoys homemade gnocchis (organic and gluten-free), wine, and good conversation. Today, her passion is healing her seven-year-old son and educating families on modern wellness. She believes anything is possible, and is known to jump in the ring when the cause is important to her. It should be no surprise that her favorite *Rocky* quote is "Going in one more round when you don't think you can— that's what makes all the difference in your life." Whether your children are newly diagnosed or you have been at it a while, always hope for more. Don't let anyone make you think otherwise.

She has presented at AutismOne with leading physicians and parents, is featured in the trailer for *Undocumented Hope*, and blogs for NobleCarriage.com.

Rogue Zebra virtually lives in her own little world, far from the African savannah. Her family's rogue adventures are of their own kind, and they started eight years ago with stroke, seizures, Asperger's, and the decision to switch to a gluten- and casein-free diet "cold turkey." Next came virtual school and real learning from the comfort and warmth of home, with the flexibility of homeschooling and structure of brick and mortar.

When not explaining the difference between momentum and inertia, RZ is involved in the undiagnosed, mitochondrial, and—occasionally—ASD communities. She thinks that the paradigm "When you hear hoofbeats, think horses, not zebras" is an outdated one that needs to change. She herself is partial to "When you hear hoofbeats, THINK."

ShamROCK: I am a mother to three beautiful children, one of whom is recovering from ASD. I am a Thinker who won't stop until my son and family are healed, and until all our "canaries in the coal mine" have returned to health. Our kids need help in their recovery. We can't do it alone. Peace, xoxo.

Shawty (Terri Burges Hirning): I am a proud mother of three children: two born to me and one I was lucky enough to get as a bonus gift through marriage. My son is recovered from autism thanks to some serious teamwork and the tireless help and support of my husband. As a result of my journey, I also work full time in the autism world helping others in a way I never dreamed possible. I also mentor and blog in my "spare" time. I am obsessed with allergen-friendly cooking, meditation, natural healing methods, crafting, gardening, sustainability, growing as much food as we can, and just trying to keep up with our children, goats, chickens, cats, and dog. I'm Wonder Woman with a generous helping of attitude and a dash of ghetto-fabulous! In response to my family's journey, I cofounded Real Food Mum in an effort to help other families transition to a real food diet: www.realfoodmum.com.

Spark (Jaima Gadeaun): I am a mama to four beautiful children, one who was diagnosed with autism and one with Tourette's. I am grateful to all those moms who have shown me the way and provided me with hope and encouragement on this journey. I believe it is time to pay it forward and provide others with the same. I am thankful for my husband, who works tirelessly so that we can afford the recovery of our girls. I'm addicted to Pinterest, paper crafts, and stamping.

Spartan (Maria O'Neil) hails from New York, where she once worked in mainstream healthcare. Since marrying her Marine husband in 2006, she has been everywhere from North Carolina to Okinawa, Japan, where her son received an autism diagnosis at eighteen months. Since recovering her son, Connor, now age five, her main focus is advocating for choices and different options in treating autism, along with keeping autism at bay in her youngest son, Cash. Marine wives are often referred to as "Spartan Wives." Historically, Spartans are brave, undaunted warriors in battle—and battle this Spartan will until every parent she meets knows that they indeed have options and can treat the medical component of today's autism.

Sunflower (Laurie Connell): I am a mom of two wonderful boys. Our youngest son is my focus, and my mission is to heal and recover him from iatrogenic autism. Each day holds amazing surprises from our sweet, smart, and funny little boy. In my former life, I had a successful twenty-year career in new home sales. Baton twirling was my passion from childhood through college. Currently, I enjoy yoga, walks with our dog, outdoor activities with the family, shopping at our local health food store, juicing, and watching HGTV. I now have a successful home-based business as an independent distributor with It Works! (www.HopeWrappedInBetterHealth.com).

We are very active in helping families newly diagnosed with autism and offering them HOPE. I am grateful for a supportive husband, family, and for all of their help. My faith as a Christian is what keeps me going, as well as the wonderful friends cheering us on.

Zorro (Jill Rege) is a California mom with a point to make about autism (and ADHD, and sensory integration dysfunction): it has biological underpinnings and is treatable! Kids can improve and some can recover when their medical issues and nutritional deficiencies are corrected. Mom to three boys with issues including anxiety, autism (her son has recovered!), ADHD, epilepsy, dyslexia, and mild attachment disorder, Zorro spends her days looking for solutions, geeking out over neurobiology, juggling schedules, trying to feed picky kids with a billion food allergies, and keeping up with celebrity gossip. She blogs at *Recovery Road* (https://recoveryrd.com/).